Atlas of Pulmonary Vascular Imaging

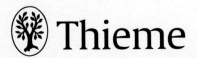

Atlas of Pulmonary Vascular Imaging

Conrad Wittram, MB, ChB
Associate Professor
Department of Radiology
Harvard Medical School
Massachusetts General Hospital
Boston, Massachusetts

Thieme
New York • Stuttgart

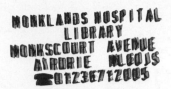
Thieme Medical Publishers, Inc.
333 Seventh Ave.
New York, NY 10001

Executive Editor: Timothy Hiscock
Managing Editor: J. Owen Zurhellen IV
Editorial Director: Michael Wachinger
Production Editor: Kenneth L. Chumbley, Publication Services
International Production Director: Andreas Schabert
Vice President, International Marketing and Sales: Cornelia Schulze
Chief Financial Officer: James W. Mitos
President: Brian D. Scanlan
Compositor: Thomson Digital
Printer: Leo Paper Group

Library of Congress Cataloging-in-Publication Data

Wittram, Conrad.
   Atlas of pulmonary vascular imaging / Conrad Wittram.
      p. ; cm.
   Includes bibliographical references.
   Summary: "Packed with detailed, clearly labeled radiologic images on every page, this lavishly illustrated atlas teaches readers how to identify and quickly diagnose the spectrum of pulmonary vascular pathologies using the full range of imaging modalities. Each concise yet comprehensive chapter provides systematic coverage of the imaging manifestations of common, uncommon, and rare diseases. Explanatory text supplements each high-quality image to highlight only the most relevant, must-know information"–Provided by publisher.
   ISBN 978-1-60406-312-7 (alk. paper)
   1. Lungs–Blood-vessels–Diseases--Atlases. I. Title.
   [DNLM: 1. Vascular Diseases–diagnosis–Atlases. 2. Diagnostic Imaging–Atlases. 3. Pulmonary Artery–physiopathology–Atlases. 4. Pulmonary Veins–physiopathology–Atlases. WG 17 W756a 2010]
   RC776.V37W58 2010
   616.2'40022--dc22
                          2010018529

Important note: Medical knowledge is ever-changing. As new research and clinical experience broaden our knowledge, changes in treatment and drug therapy may be required. The authors and editors of the material herein have consulted sources believed to be reliable in their efforts to provide information that is complete and in accord with the standards accepted at the time of publication. However, in view of the possibility of human error by the authors, editors, or publisher of the work herein or changes in medical knowledge, neither the authors, editors, nor publisher, nor any other party who has been involved in the preparation of this work, warrants that the information contained herein is in every respect accurate or complete, and they are not responsible for any errors or omissions or for the results obtained from use of such information. Readers are encouraged to confirm the information contained herein with other sources. For example, readers are advised to check the product information sheet included in the package of each drug they plan to administer to be certain that the information contained in this publication is accurate and that changes have not been made in the recommended dose or in the contraindications for administration. This recommendation is of particular importance in connection with new or infrequently used drugs.

Some of the product names, patents, and registered designs referred to in this book are in fact registered trademarks or proprietary names even though specific reference to this fact is not always made in the text. Therefore, the appearance of a name without designation as proprietary is not to be construed as a representation by the publisher that it is in the public domain.

Printed in China

5 4 3 2 1

ISBN 978-1-60406-312-7

To my family: past, present, and future.

Contents

Foreword

As computed tomography (CT) and magnetic resonance imaging (MRI) continue to improve, the depiction of the pulmonary and systemic vessels in the thorax has improved dramatically. With better spatial resolution, contrast resolution, and temporal resolution, the pulmonary vessels and their relation to other intrathoracic structures are shown in ways never possible before. This exquisite vascular detail enhances diagnoses of many congenital and acquired diseases. In this text, Wittram provides a succinct, beautifully illustrated demonstration of normal anatomy and how a detailed understanding of this anatomy aids in the diagnosis of disease and, often, in the understanding of the underlying pathophysiology.

The twelve chapters touch on a surprising number of diseases, both common and rare. The initial chapter on normal anatomy sets the stage with excellent drawings and medical images (X-ray, computed tomography, magnetic resonance imaging, and angiography). Two chapters follow on the vascular changes in congenital lung disease and cardiac disorders.

The remaining chapters focus on specific categories of disease, such as pulmonary embolism, vasculitis, pulmonary hypertension, tumor, etc. Each chapter is well-organized, with clear images and a pertinent bibliography.

This sharply focused book will be of great interest to *all* radiologists, as it gives us a greater appreciation of the increased vascular detail—available now in daily practice—and how to utilize it to arrive at better diagnosis. Pulmonologists and surgeons, who deal with these issues on a daily basis, will also find this enlightening.

Lawrence R. Goodman, MD, FACR
Professor
Department of Diagnostic Radiology and Diagnostic
Radiology and Pulmonary Medicine & Critical Care
Director
Department of Thoracic Imaging
Medical College of Wisconsin
Milwaukee, Wisconsin

Preface

Multidetector computed tomography has revolutionized the imaging of acute pulmonary embolism and ushered in a new radiology discipline: pulmonary vascular imaging. This *Atlas of Pulmonary Vascular Imaging* uses a comprehensive and systematic approach to illustrate the radiographic, angiographic, magnetic resonance, ultrasound, and nuclear medicine imaging manifestations of the new discipline, in addition to the computed tomographic imaging manifestations of common, uncommon, and quite rare diseases of pulmonary vessels.

The book has been written for physicians specializing in radiology, pulmonology, cardiology, or cardiothoracic surgery, and for residents training in these specialties. It provides a foundation of understanding and encourages interest and further research in pulmonary vascular disease. *Atlas of Pulmonary Vascular Imaging* begins with an overview of normal pulmonary vascular anatomy and common variants. The book then examines the effects of congenital anomalies, cardiac disease, emboli, in situ thrombosis, vasculitis, infections, tumors, and systemic and lung diseases on pulmonary vessels. The imaging manifestations of pulmonary vessel aneurysms and varices are reviewed, and the book concludes with a chapter on pulmonary arterial hypertension. The text is bulleted and the content concise, with only important information presented. Lists of suggested reading are provided for those who desire more in-depth information. I hope and expect that this work will prove to be stimulating and educational and that it will ultimately benefit patient care.

Acknowledgments

I owe a debt of gratitude to Sue Loomis for her outstanding efforts in creating the color drawings and preparing all the figures for publication. I also would like to acknowledge my colleagues and the countless radiology fellows, residents, and medical students whom it has been a privilege and pleasure to work with, learn from, and teach over the course of my career.

1

Anatomy

The vessels supplying the lungs include the pulmonary arteries, pulmonary veins, and bronchial arteries. In this chapter, the predominant branching patterns are illustrated and variants of the pulmonary vasculature are explored. Knowledge of variant anatomy is important as this can, occasionally, mimic disease and, when necessary, allow for correct surgical and interventional procedure planning.

◆ Pulmonary Arteries

- ◆ The main pulmonary artery arises from the right ventricle distal to the pulmonary valve and courses cephalad

and dorsally; it divides into right and left pulmonary arteries (**Figs. 1.1, 1.2, 1.3, 1.4,** and **1.5**).
- ◆ The right pulmonary artery divides into the truncus anterior (superior trunk) and the interlobar pulmonary artery.
- ◆ The left pulmonary artery supplies the upper lobe, lingula, and lower lobe of the left lung.
- ◆ In each lung, the common patterns are lobar and 10 segmental arterial structures.
- ◆ The segmental arteries are adjacent to their accompanying bronchi, situated medial to the bronchi in the upper lobes and laterally in the lingula and middle and lower lobes.
- ◆ The subsegmental arteries are identified as dichotomous divisions of the segmental arteries.

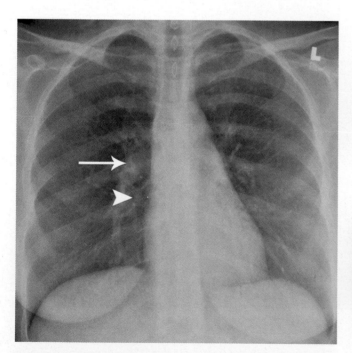

A

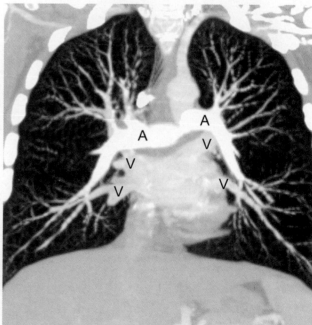

B

Fig. 1.1 (A–F) Normal chest radiographs and CT images in a 22-year-old woman. **(A)** Anteroposterior chest radiograph. The normal hila shadows are made up of pulmonary arteries and veins and bronchial walls. The right superior pulmonary vein is overlying the right interlobar artery (*arrow*). The right inferior pulmonary vein is also identified

(*arrowhead*). **(B)** Coronal reformatted CT image of the same patient demonstrates the normal hilar relationships of the right and left pulmonary arteries (*A*) and the right and left superior and inferior pulmonary veins (*V*).   (*Continued on page 2*)

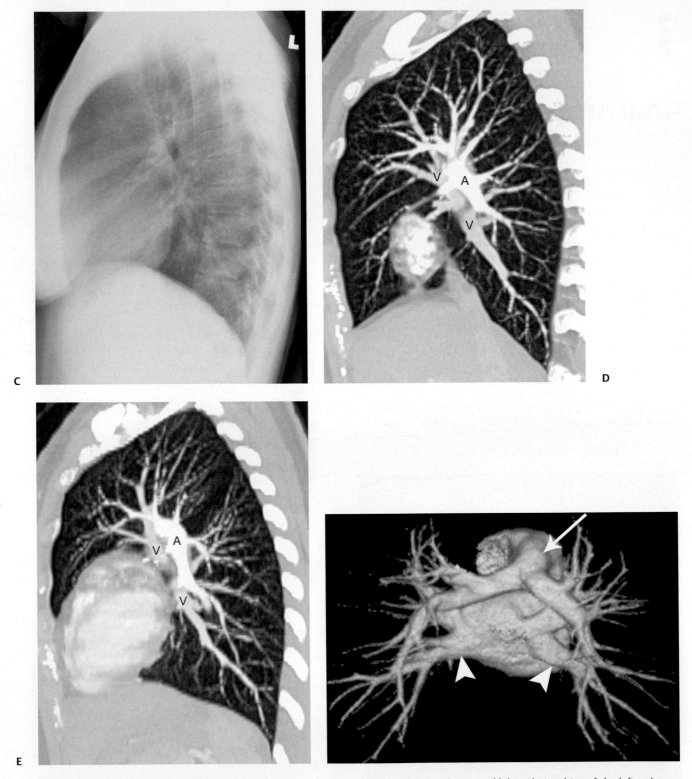

Fig. 1.1 (*Continued*) Normal chest radiographs and CT images in a 22-year-old woman. **(C)** Normal lateral radiograph has both hilar shadows superimposed to form a composite shadow, which can be difficult to interpret. **(D)** Sagittal reformatted CT image elegantly demonstrates the normal hilar relationships of the right pulmonary artery (*A*) and the right superior and right inferior pulmonary veins (*V*). **(E)** Sagittal reformatted CT image shows the normal hilar relationships of the left pulmonary artery (*A*) and the left superior and left inferior pulmonary veins (*V*). **(F)** Posterior view of a surface-rendered three-dimensional CT image demonstrates the orientation of the pulmonary arteries with respect to the pulmonary veins; the main pulmonary artery (*arrow*) and inferior pulmonary veins (*arrowheads*) are indicated.

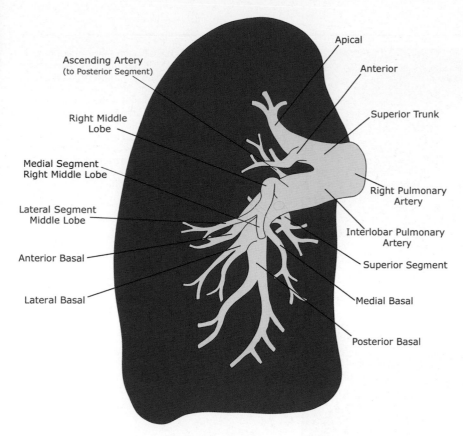

Apical

Anterior

Superior Trunk

Ascending Artery
(to Posterior Segment)

Right Middle
Lobe

Medial Segment
Right Middle Lobe

Right Pulmonary
Artery

Lateral Segment
Middle Lobe

Interlobar Pulmonary
Artery

Anterior Basal

Superior Segment

Lateral Basal

Medial Basal

Posterior Basal

Fig. 1.2 Illustration of right pulmonary artery anatomy.

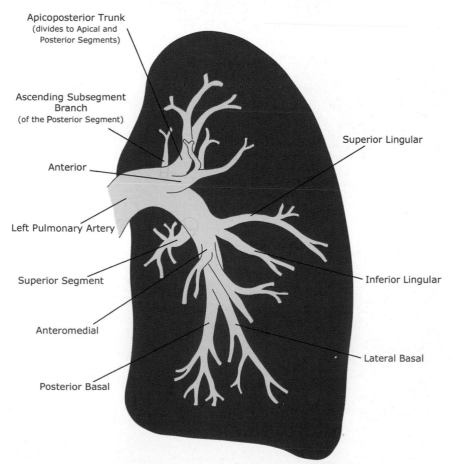

Apicoposterior Trunk
(divides to Apical and
Posterior Segments)

Ascending Subsegment
Branch
(of the Posterior Segment)

Superior Lingular

Anterior

Left Pulmonary Artery

Superior Segment

Inferior Lingular

Anteromedial

Lateral Basal

Posterior Basal

Fig. 1.3 Illustration of left pulmonary artery anatomy.

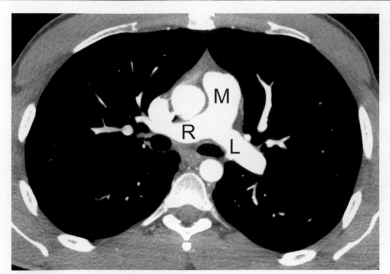

A

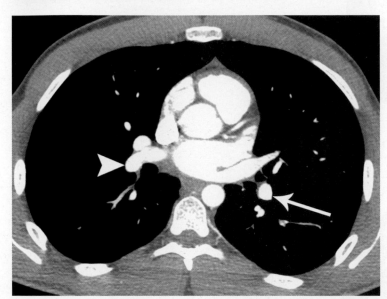

B

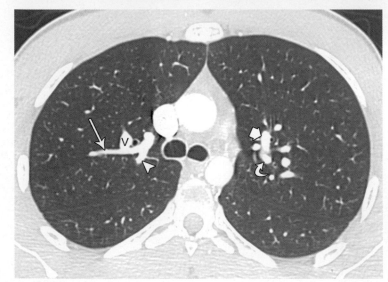

C

Fig. 1.4 (A–J) Normal axial CT pulmonary angiograms in a 22-year-old woman. **(A)** Mediastinal window settings demonstrate the normal main (*M*), right (*R*), and left (*L*) pulmonary arteries. **(B)** Image at the level of the left atrium demonstrates the normal right interlobar pulmonary artery (*arrowhead*) and left lower lobe artery (*arrow*). **(C)** Lung window settings at the level of the carina demonstrate subsegmental branches of the right upper lobe posterior artery (*arrow* and *arrowhead*) and a branch of the right superior pulmonary vein (*V*). On the left side, the apical (*short arrow*) and posterior (*curved arrow*) segmental arteries are identified.

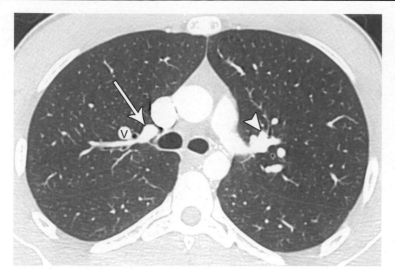

D

Fig. 1.4 (*Continued*) Normal axial CT pulmonary angiograms in a 22-year-old woman. **(D)** Image obtained slightly more caudad than the image in **C** demonstrates the right upper lobe apical segmental artery (*arrow*) and a branch of the right superior pulmonary vein (*V*), as well as the left upper lobe anterior segmental artery (*arrowhead*). **(E)** Image at the level of the main pulmonary artery demonstrates a branch of the right upper lobe anterior artery (*arrow*) and a branch of the right superior pulmonary vein (*V*). On the left side, a branch of the left lower lobe superior segmental artery (*arrowhead*) and branches of the left superior pulmonary vein (*V*) are seen. **(F)** Image at the level of the right ventricle outflow tract shows the right interlobar artery (*arrow*), right superior pulmonary vein (*V*), superior lingular segmental artery (*short arrow*), and left lower lobe artery (*arrowhead*). (*Continued on page 6*)

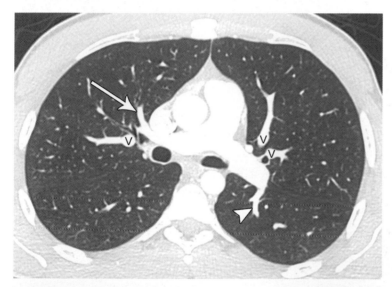

E

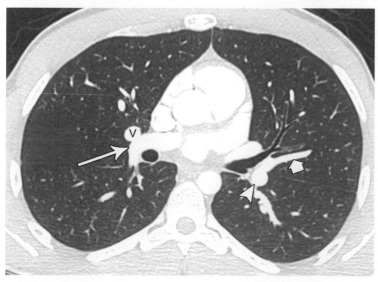

F

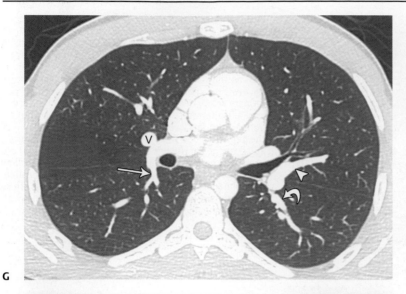

G

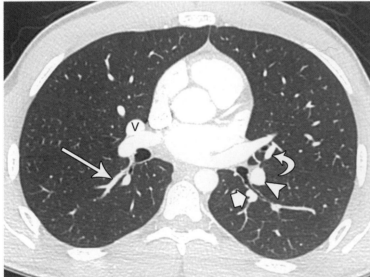

H

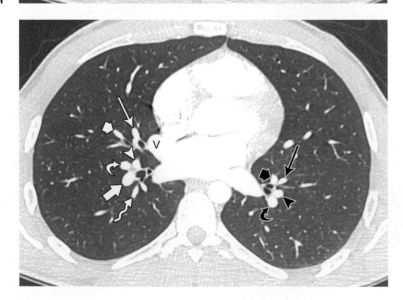

I

Fig. 1.4 (*Continued*) Normal axial CT pulmonary angiograms in a 22-year-old woman. **(G)** Image obtained slightly more caudad than the image in **F** shows the right lower lobe superior segmental artery (*arrow*), right superior pulmonary vein (*V*), lingular artery (*arrowhead*), and left lower lobe superior segmental artery (*curved arrow*). **(H)** Image at the level of the left atrium shows a branch of the right lower lobe superior segmental artery (*arrow*), the right superior pulmonary vein (*V*), the inferior lingular segmental artery (*curved arrow*), the left posterior basal segmental artery (*short arrow*), and the anteromedial-lateral basal segment trunk artery (*arrowhead*). **(I)** Image at the level of the left atrium demonstrates the right medial middle lobe segmental artery (*white long arrow*), the right lateral middle lobe segmental artery (*white short arrow*), the right medial basal segmental artery (*white arrowhead*), the right anterior basal segmental artery (*white curved arrow*), a lateral-posterior basal segment trunk artery (*white thick arrow*), and a pulmonary vein branch (*white squiggly arrow*). On the left side, the left posterior basal segment artery (*black curved arrow*) and the lateral basal segmental artery (*black arrowhead*) are seen, and the anteromedial basal segmental artery has branched into two arteries (*black long* and *short arrows*). On this image, the right superior pulmonary vein (*V*) and the right and left inferior pulmonary veins are also seen draining into the left atrium.

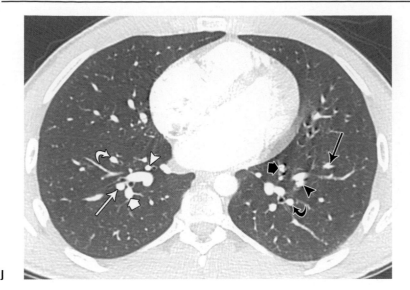

J

Fig. 1.4 (*Continued*) Normal axial CT pulmonary angiograms in a 22-year-old woman. **(J)** Image at the level of the left atrium demonstrates the right medial basal segmental artery (*white arrowhead*), right anterior basal segmental artery (*white curved arrow*), lateral basal segmental artery (*white arrow*), and right posterior basal segmental artery (*white thick arrow*). On the left side, the left posterior basal segmental artery (*black curved arrow*) and lateral basal segmental artery (*black arrowhead*) are seen, and the anteromedial basal segmental artery has branched into subsegmental arteries (*black long* and *short arrows*).

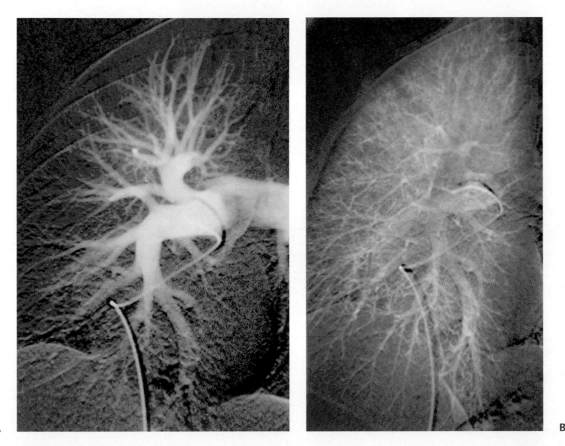

A

B

Fig. 1.5 (A–D) Normal pulmonary angiograms in a 36-year-old woman. **(A)** Right lung in arterial phase. **(B)** Right lung in capillary phase. (*Continued on page 8*)

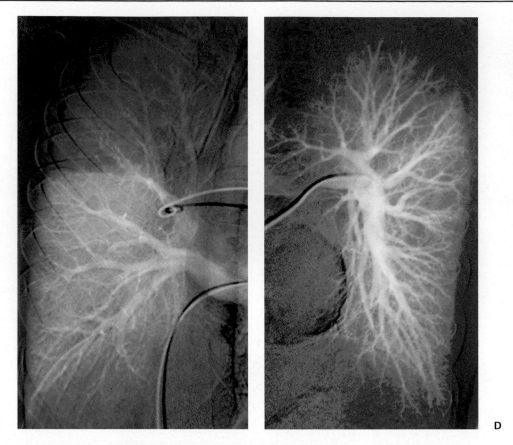

C

D

Fig. 1.5 (*Continued*) Normal pulmonary angiograms in a 36-year-old woman. **(C)** Right lung in venous phase. **(D)** Left lung in arterial phase.

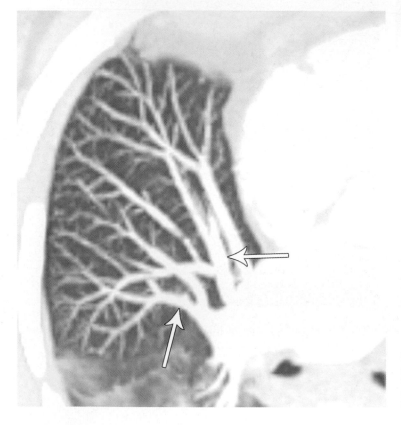

Fig. 1.6 Variant middle lobe arteries in a 53-year-old woman. Axial CT maximum-intensity projection (MIP) image demonstrates the medial and lateral segmental pulmonary arteries arising individually from the right interlobar pulmonary artery (*arrows*).

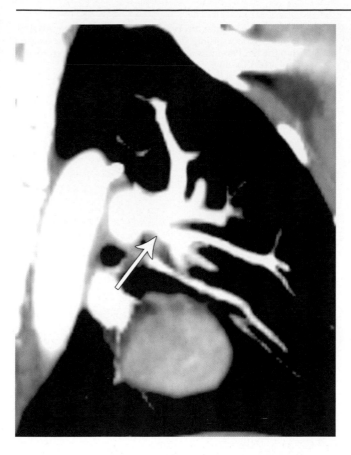

Fig. 1.7 High lingular artery in a 64-year-old man. Oblique sagittal reformatted CT image demonstrates the lingular artery arising from the left upper lobe artery (*arrow*).

Right Pulmonary Artery

♦ The right upper lobe is supplied by the truncus anterior, which gives rise to the apical and anterior segmental arteries. The posterior segment is supplied by the ascending artery from the interlobar pulmonary artery.

♦ The middle lobe artery arises from the right interlobar artery anteriorly and then branches into the medial and lateral segmental arteries. In a variant of this arrangement, the medial and lateral segments come directly from the interlobar artery (**Fig. 1.6**).

♦ The interlobar artery becomes the right lower lobe artery after giving rise to the middle lobe artery. The next branch is the superior segmental artery, which comes off the right lower lobe artery posteriorly. The lower lobe artery then gives rise to the four basal segmental arteries, which follow the bronchial divisions.

Left Pulmonary Artery

♦ The left upper lobe is supplied by an apicoposterior truncal artery, which divides into the apical and posterior segmental arteries. The anterior segmental artery comes directly off the right pulmonary artery anteriorly. There is also an ascending subsegmental branch to the posterior segment.

♦ The lingular artery arises from the pulmonary artery and divides into the superior and inferior segmental arteries. Variant origins are from the left upper lobe artery (**Fig. 1.7**) or the left lower lobe artery (**Fig. 1.8**).

♦ The superior segmental artery arises from the posterior part of the left lower lobe artery; it often then divides into anteromedial and posterolateral common trunks, the former of which subsequently divides into anterior and medial and the latter into posterior and lateral basal segmental arteries.

Normal Pulmonary Artery Diameters

♦ Since the 1970s, numerous studies with varying methodologies and patient populations have used computed tomography (CT) to measure the normal pulmonary diameters. These studies have come up with diameters ranging from 25 to 36 mm for the main pulmonary artery (**Fig. 1.9**).

♦ As an absolute figure, a main pulmonary artery diameter of more than 29 mm is widely considered enlarged and suggestive of pulmonary artery hypertension.

♦ The normal ratio of the diameter of a peripheral pulmonary artery to the diameter of the accompanying bronchus ranges from 1.0 to 1.2. Enlargement of the peripheral pulmonary arteries is a common CT finding in pulmonary artery hypertension.

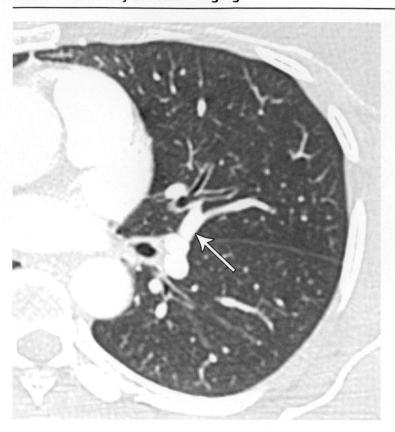

Fig. 1.8 Low lingular artery in a 47-year-old woman. Axial CT on lung window settings demonstrates a lingular artery arising from the left lower lobe artery at the level of the anteromedial basal artery (*arrow*).

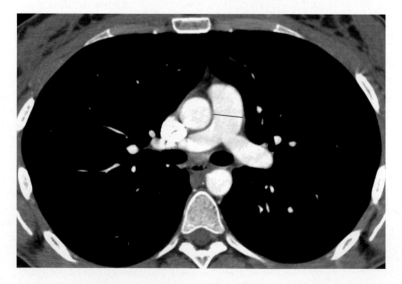

Fig. 1.9 Measurement of the main pulmonary artery in a 22-year-old woman. Axial image demonstrates the largest diameter of the main pulmonary artery. The line of the measurement is perpendicular to the vessel walls (*black line*) and in this case is 25 mm in length.

◆ Pulmonary Veins

- ◆ The veins are found in the periphery of the lung from the level of the secondary pulmonary lobule to the levels of the subsegments, segments, and lobes.
- ◆ Right superior and inferior pulmonary veins and left superior and inferior pulmonary veins drain directly into the left atrium (**Figs. 1.1, 1.4, 1.10, 1.11, and 1.12**).
- ◆ The right superior pulmonary vein drains the right upper lobe and right middle lobe.
- ◆ The right inferior pulmonary vein drains the right lower lobe.
- ◆ The left superior pulmonary vein drains the left upper lobe and lingula.
- ◆ The left inferior pulmonary vein drains the left lower lobe.
- ◆ Pulmonary vein diameters are typically reduced in patients with precapillary pulmonary artery hyperten-sion and enlarged in those with raised left atrial pressure.

Right Pulmonary Veins

- ◆ The right upper lobe apical, anterior, and posterior veins combine to form a trunk anterior to the right interlobar artery.
- ◆ The middle lobe lateral and medial veins combine to form a medial lobe trunk. This joins the upper lobe vein to form the right superior pulmonary vein, which then enters the left atrium.
- ◆ The anterior, posterior, medial, and lateral basal segmen-tal veins combine to form a trunk. This joins the superior vein (draining the superior segment of the lower lobe) to form the right inferior pulmonary vein, which then enters the left atrium (**Fig. 1.10**).

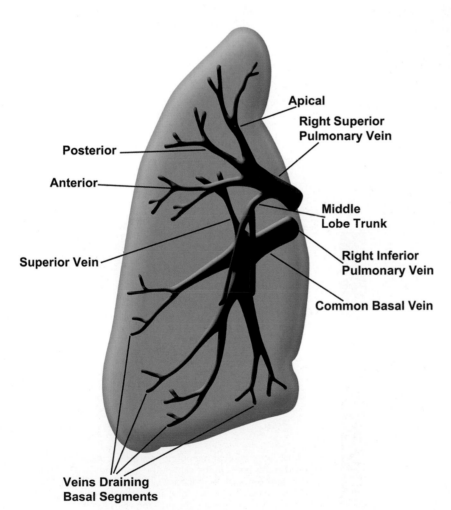

Fig. 1.10 Illustration of the right pulmonary veins.

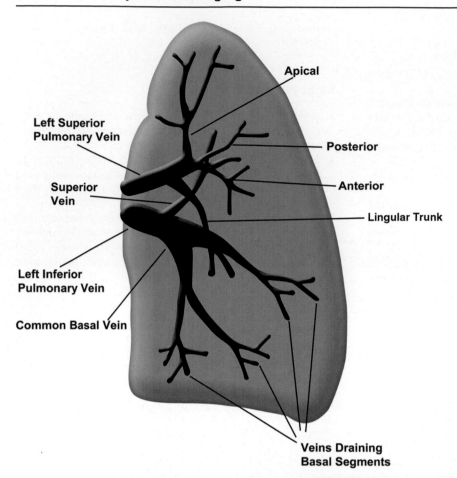

Fig. 1.11 Illustration of the left pulmonary veins.

Apical

Left Superior
Pulmonary Vein

Posterior

Anterior

Superior
Vein

Lingular Trunk

Left Inferior
Pulmonary Vein

Common Basal Vein

Veins Draining
Basal Segments

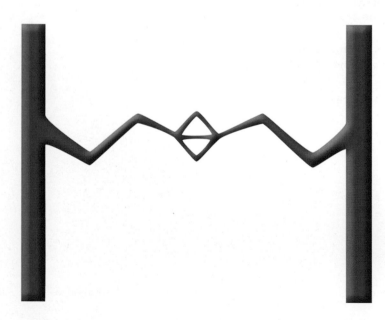

Fig. 1.12 Illustration of the pulmonary artery, veins, and capillaries used in this book. In the center, the diamond shape with a line across represents the pulmonary capillaries; to the right of the capillaries are the subsegmental and segmental arteries, and to the left of the capillaries are the draining veins.

Left Pulmonary Veins

- The left upper lobe apical, anterior, and posterior veins combine to form a trunk anterior to the left pulmonary artery.
- The superior and inferior lingular veins combine to form a trunk. This joins the upper lobe vein to form the left superior pulmonary vein, which then enters the left atrium.
- The anteromedial, posterior, and lateral basal segmental veins combine to form a trunk. This joins the superior vein (draining the superior segment of the lower lobe) to form the left inferior pulmonary vein, which then enters the left atrium (**Fig. 1.11**).

Variant Pulmonary Vein Anatomy

- The right upper lobe posterior segmental vein, instead of running anterior to the interlobar artery, can run behind the bronchus intermedius (**Fig. 1.13**). This vein often joins the right inferior pulmonary vein and sometimes joins the left atrium directly.
- The middle lobe vein on occasion drains into the right inferior pulmonary vein (**Fig. 1.14**) or directly into the left atrium (**Fig. 1.15**).
- Similarly, the lingular vein can drain into the left inferior pulmonary vein (**Fig. 1.16**).
- A single left (or right) pulmonary vein can form and then enter the left atrium through a single ostium. Similarly, under-incorporation of the two superior veins or two inferior veins can occur. The condition in which all four vessels connect to a common chamber opening into the left atrium is known as cor triatrium.

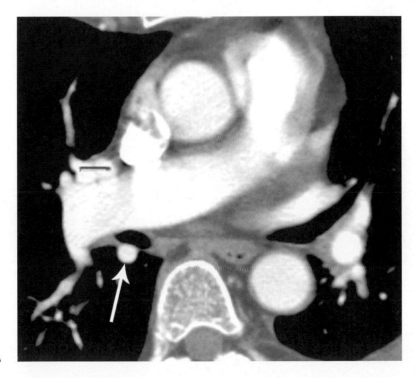

A

Fig. 1.13 (A,B) Variant right upper lobe posterior pulmonary vein in a 49-year-old women. **(A)** CT image demonstrates the right upper lobe posterior segmental vein posterior to the bronchus intermedius (*arrow*). (*Continued on page 14*)

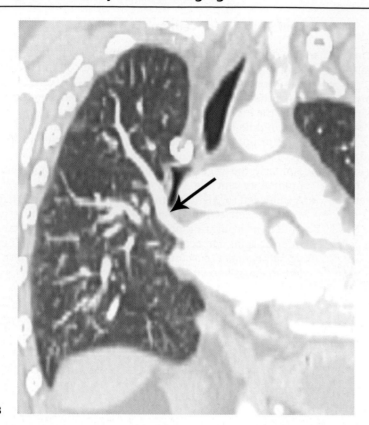

Fig. 1.13 (*Continued*) Variant right upper lobe posterior pulmonary vein in a 49-year-old woman. **(B)** Oblique coronal reformatted MIP image demonstrates the vein draining directly into the left atrium (*arrow*).

B

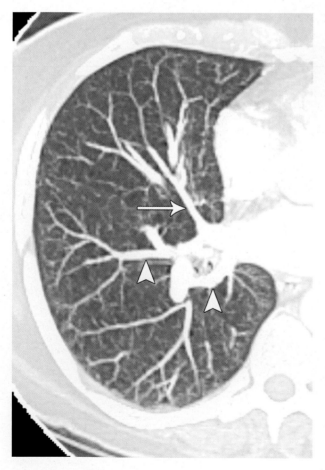

Fig. 1.14 Variant middle lobe vein in a 51-year-old man. Axial CT MIP image demonstrates middle lobe vein (*arrow*) draining into venous branches of the right lower lobe (*arrowheads*) to form the right inferior pulmonary vein.

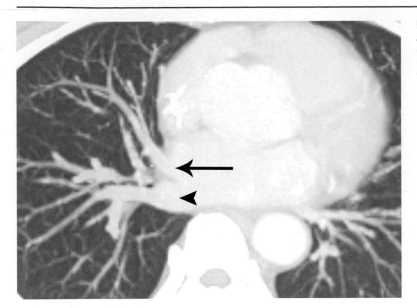

Fig. 1.15 Variant middle lobe vein in a 69-year-old man. Axial CT MIP image on lung window settings demonstrates a middle lobe vein draining directly into the left atrium (*arrow*). The right inferior pulmonary vein is demonstrated entering the left atrium more posteriorly (*arrowhead*).

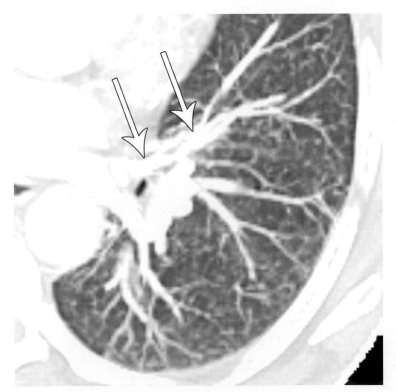

Fig. 1.16 Variant lingular vein in a 72-year-old woman. Axial CT MIP image demonstrates the lingular vein draining into the left inferior pulmonary vein (*arrows*).

◆ Bronchial Arteries

- The bronchial arteries arise from the descending thoracic aorta at the level of the left main bronchus and supply the trachea, bronchi, esophagus, and lymph nodes.
- The most common branching pattern of the bronchial arteries (type 1) consists of a single right bronchial artery arising from an intercostobronchial trunk and two left bronchial arteries (**Fig. 1.17**).
- The next most common presentation (type 2) consists of one intercostobronchial trunk on the right and one artery on the left (**Fig. 1.17**).

- An equally common pattern (type 3) consists of two arteries on the right (one intercostobronchial trunk and a right bronchial artery) and two left bronchial arteries (**Fig. 1.17**).
- The least common pattern (type 4) consists of two arteries on the right (one intercostobronchial trunk and a right bronchial artery) and one left bronchial artery (**Fig. 1.17**).
- The right intercostobronchial trunk is the most consistently identified vessel at angiography (**Fig. 1.18**). It arises from the right posterolateral part of the aorta. The right and left bronchial arteries arise from the anterolateral aspect of the aorta.

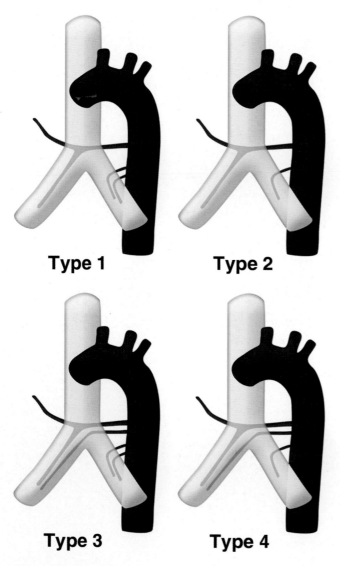

Fig. 1.17 Illustration of the common bronchial artery patterns.

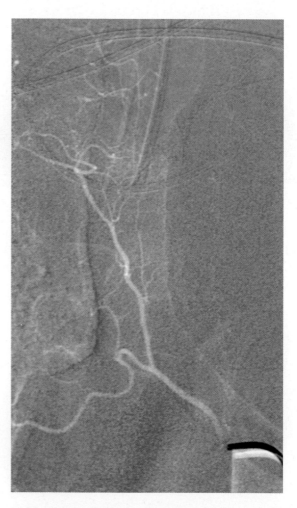

Fig. 1.18 Normal selective digital bronchial artery angiogram in a 27-year-old man. The right intercostobronchial artery branches to the right bronchus and extends superiorly to the right ribs.

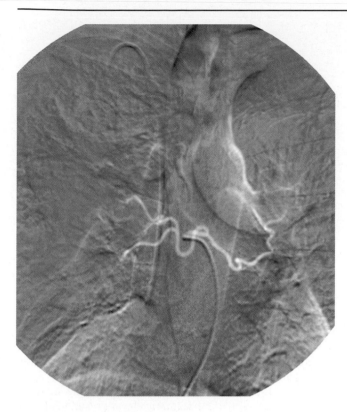

Fig. 1.19 Normal selective digital bronchial artery angiogram in a 36-year-old woman. A common origin of the right and left bronchial arteries is demonstrated, with bronchial arteries supplying both the right and left bronchi.

♦ The right and left bronchial arteries occasionally arise as a common trunk from the anterior wall of the descending thoracic aorta (**Fig. 1.19**).

♦ Bronchial arteries not arising from the descending aorta at the level of T5 and T6 are considered aberrant. Possible origins include the aortic arch, internal mammary artery, thyrocervical trunk, subclavian artery, costocervical trunk, brachiocephalic artery, pericardiacophrenic artery, inferior phrenic artery, and abdominal aorta.

♦ Normal bronchial arteries measure less than 1.5 mm in diameter at their origin. A vessel with a diameter larger than 1.5 mm is considered abnormal.

Suggested Reading

Cory RA, Valentine EJ. Varying patterns of the lobar branches of the pulmonary artery. A study of 524 lungs and lobes seen at operation of 426 patients. Thorax 1959;14:267–280

Edwards PD, Bull RK, Coulden R. CT measurement of main pulmonary artery diameter. Br J Radiol 1998;71(850):1018–1020

Ghaye B, Szapiro D, Dacher JN, et al. Percutaneous ablation for atrial fibrillation: the role of cross-sectional imaging. Radiographics 2003; 23(Spec No):S19–S33, discussion S48–S50

Guthaner DF, Wexler L, Harell G. CT demonstration of cardiac structures. AJR Am J Roentgenol 1979;133(1):75–81

Haimovici JB, Trotman-Dickenson B, Halpern EF, et al; Massachusetts General Hospital Lung Transplantation Program. Relationship between pulmonary artery diameter at computed tomography and pulmonary artery pressures at right-sided heart catheterization. Acad Radiol 1997;4(5):327–334

Jackson CL, Huber JF. Correlated applied anatomy of the bronchial tree and lungs with a system of nomenclature. Dis Chest 1943;9:319–326

Kuriyama K, Gamsu G, Stern RG, Cann CE, Herfkens RJ, Brundage BH. CT-determined pulmonary artery diameters in predicting pulmonary hypertension. Invest Radiol 1984;19(1):16–22

Schmidt HC, Kauczor HU, Schild HH, et al. Pulmonary hypertension in patients with chronic pulmonary thromboembolism: chest radiograph and CT evaluation before and after surgery. Eur Radiol 1996;6(6):817–825

Tan RT, Kuzo R, Goodman LR, Siegel R, Haasler GB, Presberg KW; Medical College of Wisconsin Lung Transplant Group. Utility of CT scan evaluation for predicting pulmonary hypertension in patients with parenchymal lung disease. Chest 1998;113(5):1250–1256

Yoon W, Kim JK, Kim YH, Chung TW, Kang HK. Bronchial and nonbronchial systemic artery embolization for life-threatening hemoptysis: a comprehensive review. Radiographics 2002;22(6):1395–1409

2

Congenital Anomalies

Congenital anomalies of the pulmonary vasculature are often asymptomatic but can present in the neonatal period or later in life. The pulmonary artery can be affected by proximal interruption (agenesis, hypoplasia, stenosis) or anomalous origin (pulmonary artery sling, truncus arteriosus). The pulmonary arterial and venous systems can have abnormal connections, as exemplified by arteriovenous malformations. An abnormal systemic artery may supply normal or abnormal lung (intralobar and extralobar sequestration, scimitar syndrome); also, abnormal systemic artery–to–pulmonary vessel shunts can occur. The pulmonary veins can be affected by a partial or total anomalous venous return draining normal or abnormal lung. In this chapter, examples are used to illustrate the numerous varied and interesting congenital anomalies of the pulmonary vasculature.

◆ Pulmonary Artery Agenesis

- ◆ Complete unilateral pulmonary artery agenesis is an uncommon anomaly that occurs on the right more often than the left.

- ◆ The affected lung is often hypoplastic and can be absent.
- ◆ The affected lung is supplied by systemic arterial blood through collaterals, mainly from bronchial arteries but also transpleural branches of the intercostal, internal mammary, subclavian, and innominate arteries.
- ◆ Left pulmonary artery agenesis is often associated with a right aortic arch and other congenital cardiovascular anomalies.
- ◆ Some patients remain asymptomatic, but recurrent pulmonary infection, hemoptysis, dyspnea on exertion, and pulmonary hypertension are seen.
- ◆ Imaging typically shows volume loss of the affected hemithorax, with diaphragmatic elevation and mediastinal shift to the affected side (**Figs. 2.1** and **2.2**); the contralateral lung is hyperinflated. Collateral vessels are often seen (**Fig. 2.1**).
- ◆ Partial unilateral pulmonary artery agenesis can also occur (**Fig. 2.3**).

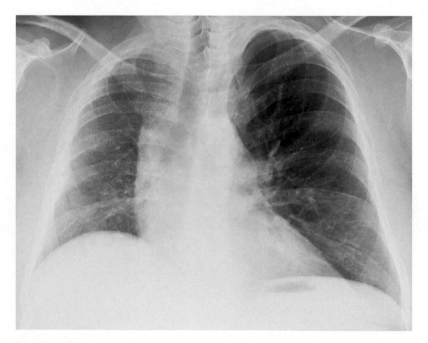

A

Fig. 2.1 (A–C) Agenesis of the right pulmonary artery in a 38-year-old man. **(A)** Chest radiograph demonstrates shift of the mediastinum to the right and a hypoplastic right lung with attenuation of the pulmonary vessels on the right.

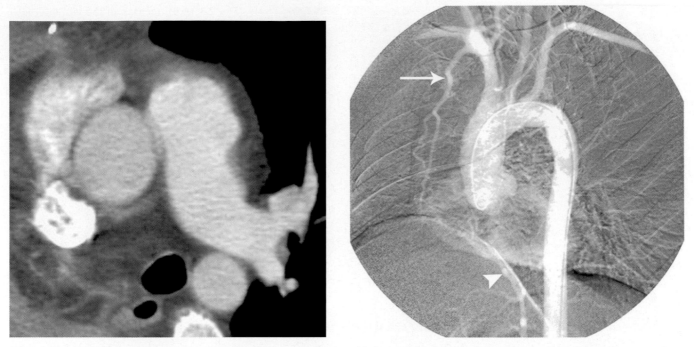

B

C

Fig. 2.1 (*Continued*) Agenesis of the right pulmonary artery in a 38-year-old man. **(B)** CT demonstrates agenesis of the right pulmonary artery. **(C)** Digital subtraction arch arteriogram demonstrates hypertrophic right internal mammary (*arrow*) and right phrenic (*arrowhead*) arteries.

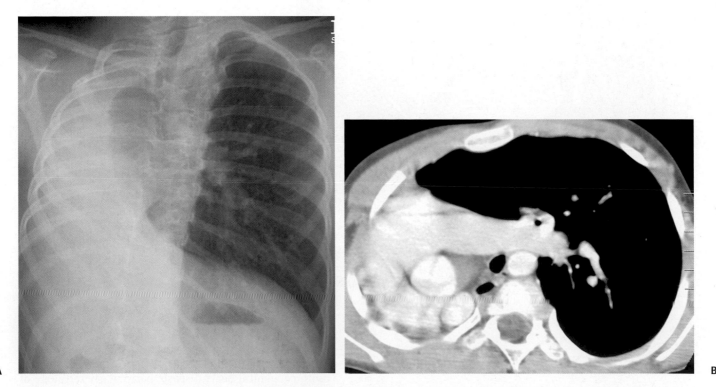

A

B

Fig. 2.2 (A,B) Agenesis of the right lung in a 7-year-old boy. **(A)** Chest radiograph demonstrates complete shift of the mediastinum to the right as the right pulmonary artery and lung did not form. **(B)** CT shows the heart against the right side of the chest wall and compensatory over-inflation of the left lung.

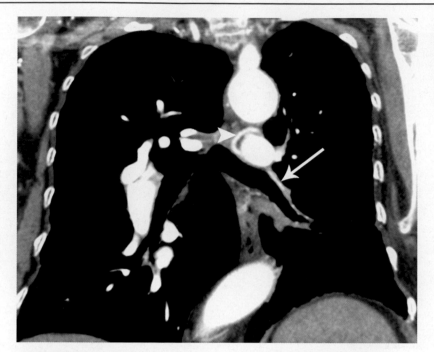

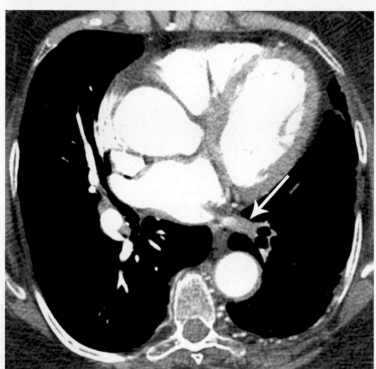

Fig. 2.3 (A,B) Agenesis of the left lower lobe pulmonary artery in a 64-year-old woman. **(A)** Coronal reformatted CT demonstrates absence of the left lower lobe pulmonary artery (*arrow*). There are collateral bronchial arteries (*arrowhead*). **(B)** A small left inferior pulmonary vein demonstrates poorly opacified pulmonary venous return (*arrow*).

◆ Pulmonary Artery Hypoplasia

◆ A unilateral congenital small pulmonary artery usually occurs in association with an ipsilateral congenital small lung (**Fig. 2.4**) because normal pulmonary blood flow is needed for normal lung development.

◆ Bilateral small pulmonary arteries are usually associated with congenital heart disease, particularly tetralogy of Fallot.

◆ The morphologic features of tetralogy of Fallot include subpulmonary infundibular stenosis, ventricular septal defect, overriding of the aorta, and right ventricular hypertrophy.

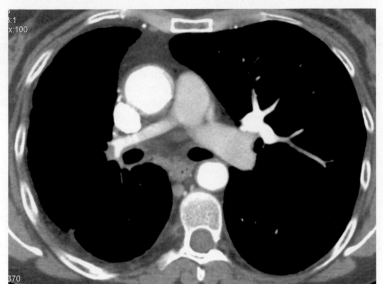

A

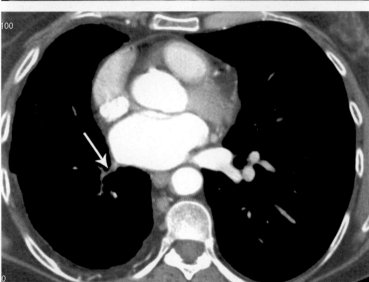

B

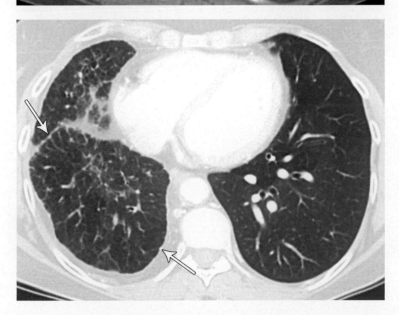

C

Fig. 2.4 (A–C) Hypoplasia of the pulmonary artery in a 40-year-old woman. **(A)** CT demonstrates a very small right pulmonary artery in comparison with the left. **(B)** CT obtained more caudad demonstrates a hypogenic right inferior pulmonary vein (*arrow*). **(C)** Lung windows at the level of the lung bases demonstrate nodularity along the pleural margins, likely due to transpleural collateral vessels (*arrows*).

◆ Pulmonary Artery Stenosis

- ◆ Pulmonary artery stenosis can be associated with other congenital cardiac malformations, as in Williams syndrome, or may occur as a primary isolated condition (**Fig. 2.5**).

◆ Left Pulmonary Artery Sling

- ◆ An aberrant left pulmonary artery arises from the proximal right pulmonary artery, courses between the trachea and esophagus, and extends to the left hilum (**Fig. 2.6**).
- ◆ Affected patients may be classified generally into two groups. Those in one group have a normal bronchial pattern; those in the other have tracheobronchial

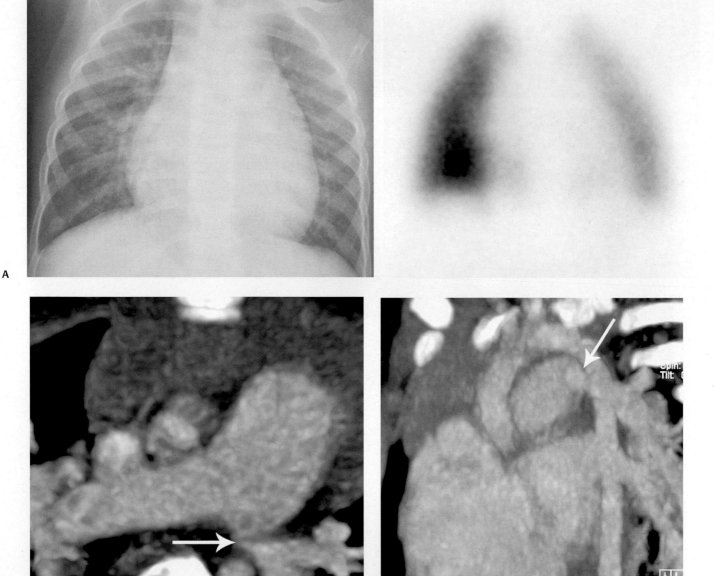

Fig. 2.5 (A–D) Pulmonary artery stenosis in an 18-month-old boy. **(A)** Chest radiograph demonstrates cardiomegaly as well as plethoric vasculature on the right. **(B)** Nuclear medicine perfusion scan demonstrates a decrease in perfusion in the left lung. **(C)** CT demonstrates a left pulmonary artery stenosis (*arrow*). **(D)** Sagittal oblique maximum-intensity projection (MIP) CT reconstruction image demonstrates the stenosis at the origin of the left pulmonary artery (*arrow*).

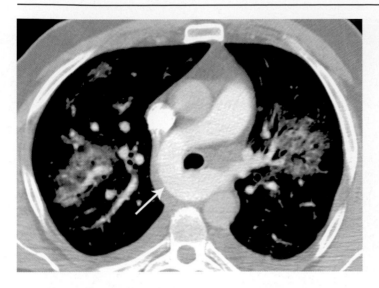

Fig. 2.6 Pulmonary artery sling in a 45-year-old man. The main pulmonary artery (*arrow*) passes to the right of the esophagus before dividing into the right and left pulmonary arteries. Lung and pleural changes of congestive heart failure are present.

malformations, including stenosis of a long segment of the trachea or absence of the pars membranacea, as well as cardiovascular abnormalities.

◆ Patients with tracheobronchial malformations have high morbidity and mortality rates during infancy.

◆ Patients without tracheobronchial malformations are often asymptomatic. The left pulmonary artery sling can mimic a mediastinal mass on chest radiography.

◆ Truncus Arteriosus

◆ Truncus arteriosus is a consequence of failure of formation of the spiral septum of the primitive truncus.

◆ Affected individuals present with a cyanotic heart lesion and increased pulmonary blood flow in the neonatal period.

◆ The single arterial trunk arises from the ventricle via a single arterial valve with two to six cusps and supplies the systemic, pulmonary, and coronary artery circulations.

◆ All patients have a high ventricular septal defect and 35% have a right aortic arch.

◆ Truncus arteriosus is classified into four types, depending on where the pulmonary arteries arise. In type 1, a short main pulmonary artery arises from the truncus; in type 2, right and left pulmonary arteries arise from the truncus posteriorly; in type 3, right and left pulmonary arteries arise from the truncus laterally; in type 4, right and left pulmonary arteries arise from the descending aorta.

◆ Imaging demonstrates enlargement of the heart and aorta (**Fig. 2.7**), often with increased pulmonary vasculature and occasionally edema.

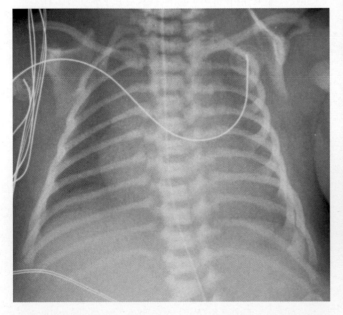

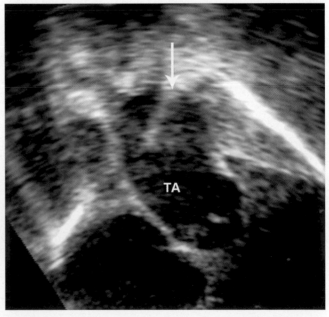

A

B

Fig. 2.7 (A–C) Truncus arteriosus in a neonate. **(A)** Chest radiograph demonstrates cardiomegaly as well as superior mediastinal fullness, consistent with a truncus arteriosus, with normal-appearing lungs and pleural spaces. **(B)** Echocardiogram demonstrates a truncus arteriosus (TA) with an echogenic septum (*arrow*). (*Continued on page 24*)

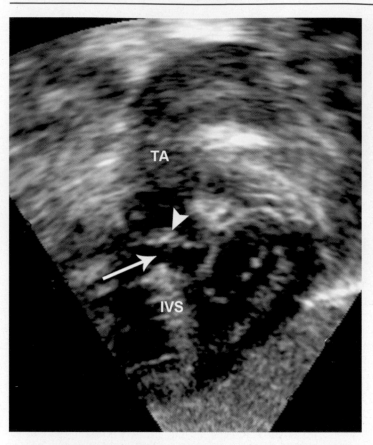

C

Fig. 2.7 (*Continued*) Truncus arteriosus in a neonate. **(C)** The truncus arteriosus (*TA*) is seen to be overlying a truncal valve (*arrowhead*); the truncal valve overlies a ventricular septal defect (*arrow*), which is superficial to the interventricular septum (*IVS*). ([**B,C**] Courtesy of David McCarty, M.D.)

◆ Pulmonary Arteriovenous Malformation

- ◆ Pulmonary arteriovenous malformations may occur in isolation, be multiple, or be part of a systemic process in which congenital arteriovenous shunts occur in the skin, mucous membranes, and other organs (hereditary hemorrhagic telangiectasia or Rendu-Osler-Weber disease).

- ◆ Acquired pulmonary arteriovenous malformations can be seen in chronic liver disease, pulmonary hypertension, systemic vein–to–pulmonary artery anastomoses, infection, and trauma.
- ◆ Imaging helps to confirm the diagnosis by demonstrating an abnormal communication between the pulmonary artery and pulmonary vein (**Figs. 2.8, 2.9,** and **2.10**).

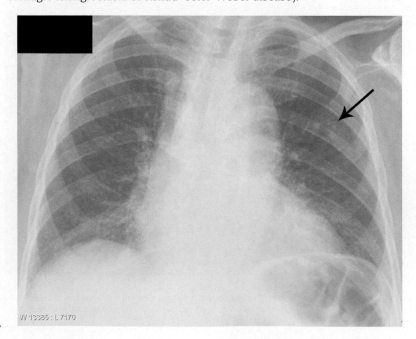

A

Fig. 2.8 (A–C) Arteriovenous malformation in an 83-year-old woman. **(A)** Chest radiograph demonstrates a serpinginous opacity overlying the left upper lobe (*arrow*).

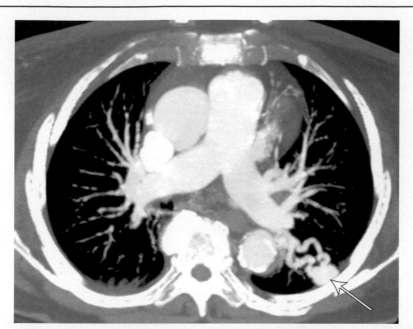

Fig. 2.8 (*Continued*) Arteriovenous malformation in an 83-year-old woman. **(B)** MIP CT demonstrates a peripheral abnormality consistent with an arteriovenous malformation (*arrow*). **(C)** Curved reformatted CT image demonstrates that the abnormality (*arrow*) is fed directly from a branch of the pulmonary artery (*PA*) and drains directly into the left atrium (*LA*), proving that it is an arteriovenous malformation.

B

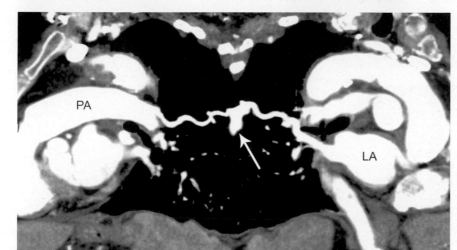

C

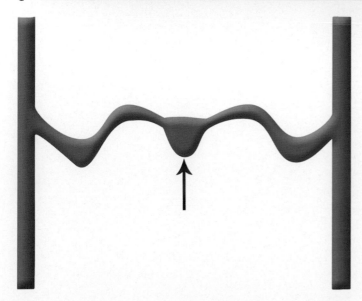

Fig. 2.9 Illustration demonstrates an arteriovenous malformation (*arrow*) with an enlarged feeding artery and a large draining vein.

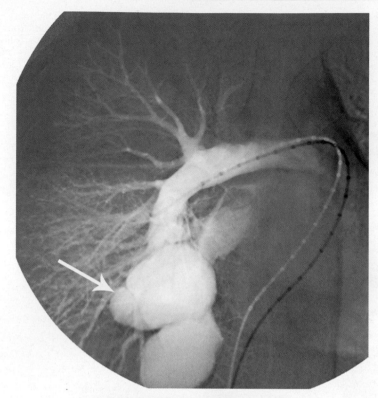

A

Fig. 2.10 (A,B) Arteriovenous malformation in a 23-year-old woman. **(A)** Pulmonary angiogram demonstrates a large arteriovenous malformation within the right lower lobe (*arrow*). **(B)** Treatment requires the use of an upstream balloon (*arrow*) to stop the arterial flow before the deployment of coils (*arrowhead*).

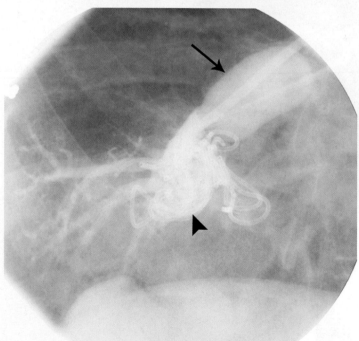

B

- ◆ Patients have a higher risk for cerebral vascular accident as a consequence of the pulmonary right-to-left shunt.
- ◆ Larger shunts can cause heart failure. This can be prevented with interventional closure (**Fig. 2.10**).

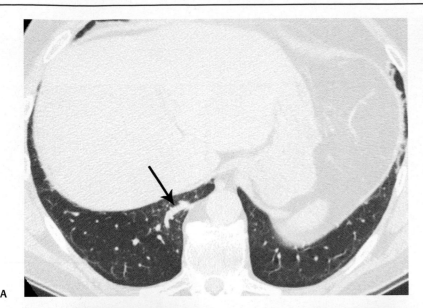

A

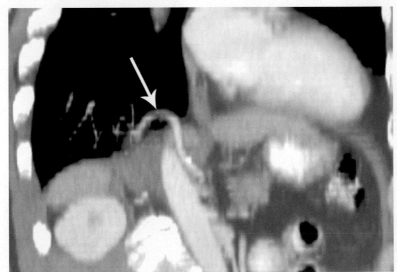

B

Fig. 2.11 (A,B) Anomalous right lower lobe pulmonary artery in a 65-year-old man. **(A)** CT on lung windows demonstrates an abnormal vessel adjacent to the vertebral column (*arrow*). **(B)** An oblique sagittal reformatted CT image shows that the systemic artery arises from the abdominal aorta (*arrow*).

◆ Systemic Artery to Normal Lung

◆ An anomalous systemic artery may supply an area of otherwise normal lung in the absence of congenital heart and lung disease (**Fig. 2.11**).

◆ It is believed that persistence of an embryonic connection between the aorta and the pulmonary parenchyma leads to this anomaly.

◆ The basal segments of the lower lobes are most often affected, more often on the left than the right.

◆ There is absence of the pulmonary artery to the affected basal segments.

◆ The involved lung has normal bronchial anatomy.

◆ Venous return is via the pulmonary vein into the left atrium.

◆ Most adult patients are asymptomatic, but some have recurrent hemoptysis.

◆ Intralobar Sequestration

◆ An anomalous systemic artery supplies an area of abnormal lung, usually at the lung base, and is surrounded by visceral pleura.

◆ Venous return is via the inferior pulmonary vein into the left atrium.

◆ There is no pulmonary artery supply to the abnormal lung.

◆ Bronchi are often absent in the abnormal lung.

◆ Intralobar sequestration often presents in adulthood without associated congenital abnormalities.

◆ Imaging demonstrates an area of increased opacity simulating pneumonia, or as a mass with or without air-fluid levels or as cysts (**Fig. 2.12**).

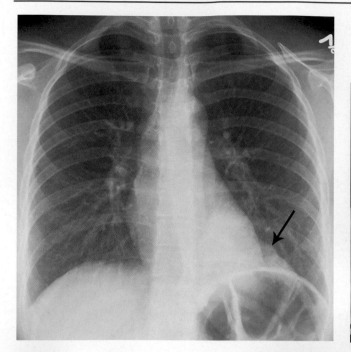

A

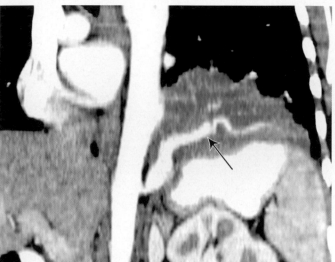

B

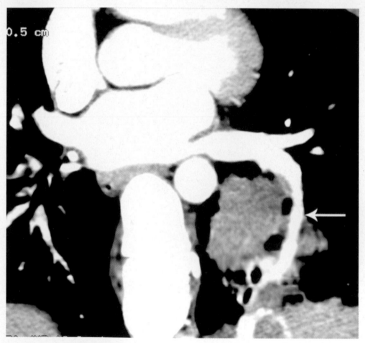

C

Fig. 2.12 (A–C) Intralobar sequestration in a 23-year-old woman. **(A)** Chest radiograph demonstrates a slightly lobulated triangular opacity extending behind the heart (*arrow*). **(B)** Curved reformatted CT image shows that the arterial supply is from the abdominal aorta (*arrow*). **(C)** Curved reformatted CT image demonstrates that the venous drainage is into the left atrium via the left inferior pulmonary vein (*arrow*).

◆ Extralobar Sequestration

- An anomalous systemic artery supplies an area of abnormal lung, usually at the lung base, with its own pleural cover. It occurs most often on the left side and can be associated with a posterior congenital diaphragmatic hernia.
- Venous return is via an abnormal systemic vein that drains via the azygos or hemiazygos veins.

- Pulmonary artery supply to the abnormal lung may be present.
- The bronchi in the abnormal lung may connect to the gastrointestinal tract.
- Extralobar sequestration presents in the neonate and is often associated with congenital heart disease.
- Imaging often demonstrates a well-defined mass at the base of the left hemithorax (**Fig. 2.13**).

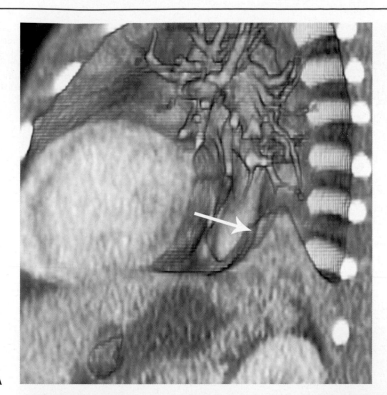

A

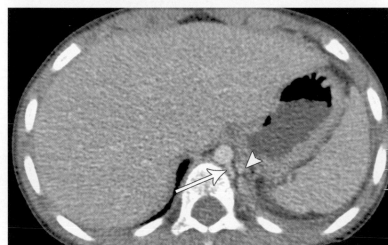

B

Fig. 2.13 (A,B) Extralobar sequestration in a neonate. **(A)** Surface-shaded coronal reformatted CT image demonstrates a smooth-margined, triangular mass in intimate contact with the left hemidiaphragm (*arrow*). **(B)** The axial contrast material–enhanced CT image demonstrates that the arterial supply is directly from the aorta (*arrow*) and that the venous drainage is to the hemiazygos vein (*arrowhead*).

◆ Hypogenetic Lung (Scimitar) Syndrome

◆ An anomalous systemic artery supplies an area of abnormal lung, usually at the right lung base, and can be associated with eventration or a diaphragmatic defect.

◆ Venous return is usually into the inferior vena cava below the right hemidiaphragm (scimitar vein), but it may be into the suprahepatic portion of the inferior vena cava, hepatic vein, portal vein, azygos vein, coronary sinus, or right atrium.

◆ Pulmonary artery supply to the abnormal lung is small or absent.

◆ Bronchial abnormalities are common, with diverticula and left bronchial isomerism.

◆ Associated cardiovascular anomalies are frequent.

◆ The presentation ranges from a neonate in heart failure to an asymptomatic adult.

◆ Imaging often demonstrates a well-defined mass at the base of the right hemithorax (**Fig. 2.14**).

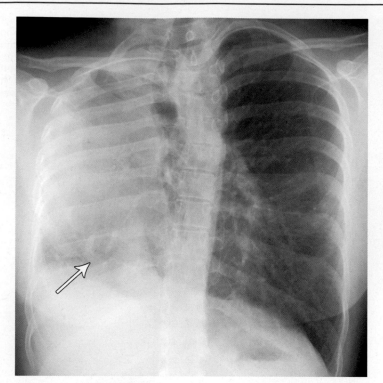

A

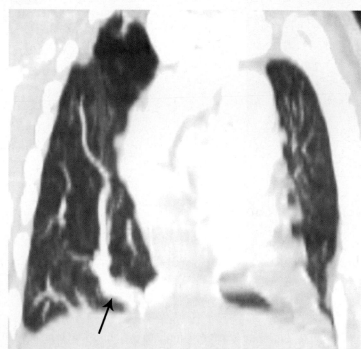

B

Fig. 2.14 (A–D) Scimitar syndrome in a 35-year-old woman. **(A)** On the chest radiograph, there is shift of the mediastinum to the right as well as a raised right hemidiaphragm, indicating volume loss. The arcuate partial anomalous pulmonary venous connection is seen heading toward the right hemidiaphragm (*arrow*). **(B)** CT coronal reconstruction MIP image shows the scimitar vein connecting to the inferior vena cava (*arrow*).

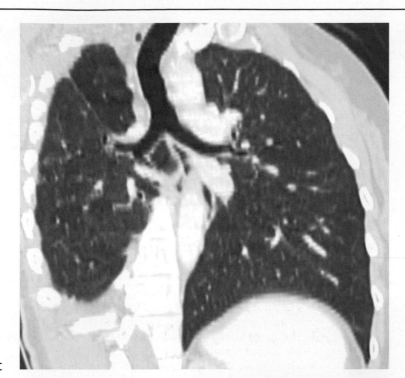

C

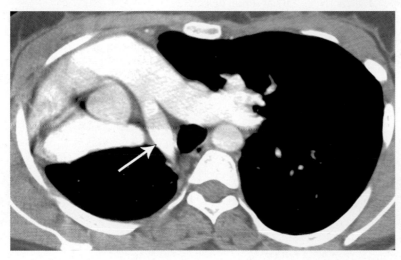

D

Fig. 2.14 (*Continued*) Scimitar syndrome in a 35-year-old woman. **(C)** CT coronal reconstruction MIP image demonstrates the abnormal bronchial anatomy on the right side. **(D)** Axial CT image demonstrates right pulmonary artery hypoplasia (*arrow*).

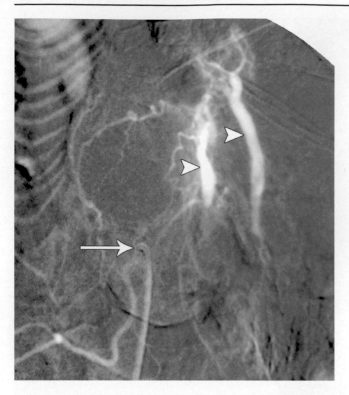

Fig. 2.15 Bronchial artery–to–pulmonary vein shunt in a 56-year-old man with hemoptysis. The catheter is within a bronchial artery (*arrow*), and the contrast material is seen to communicate with and collect within branches of the pulmonary vein of the left upper lobe (*arrowheads*).

◆ Bronchial Arteriovenous Malformation

- ◆ Bronchial arteriovenous malformation is a rare congenital disease characterized by anomalous communication between the bronchial artery and the pulmonary artery or pulmonary vein (**Fig. 2.15**).
- ◆ In 4% of all congenital pulmonary arteriovenous malformations, a feeder artery arises from the systemic circulation.
- ◆ Secondary arteriovenous malformations may be due to inflammatory lung disease or pulmonary neoplasm. A congenital lesion is thus a diagnosis of exclusion.
- ◆ Patients may be asymptomatic or present with potentially life-threatening or recurrent hemoptysis.

◆ Partial Anomalous Pulmonary Venous Return

- ◆ The pulmonary vein or veins from some portions of one or both lungs show an anomalous connection.
- ◆ The usual sites of anomalous venous return connection are the superior vena cava and the right atrium.
- ◆ There is an association with the sinus venosus type of atrial septal defect.
- ◆ The connection of the right pulmonary vein to the inferior vena cava is known as scimitar vein because of the curved shape resembling a Turkish or Arabic sword.
- ◆ An anomalous vein can appear as a band on chest radiography or be coincidentally found on computed tomography (CT) (**Fig. 2.16**).

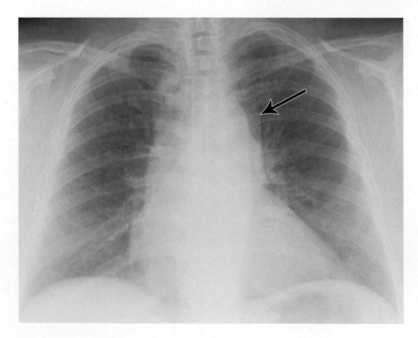

A

Fig. 2.16 (A–C) Partial anomalous pulmonary venous connection in a 37-year-old man. **(A)** Chest radiograph demonstrates a well-defined subtle opacity lateral to the aortic arch (*arrow*).

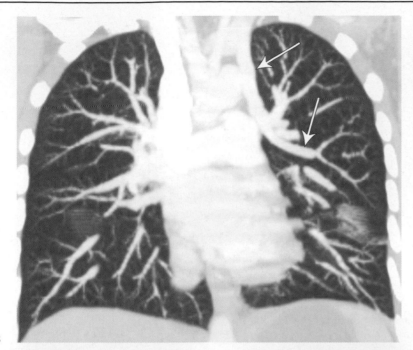

B

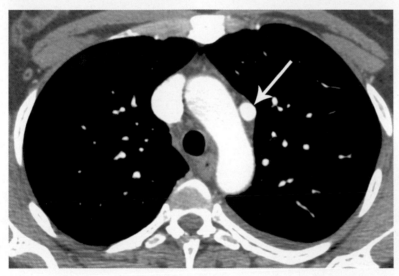

C

Fig. 2.16 (*Continued*) Partial anomalous pulmonary venous connection in a 37-year-old man. (**B**) CT coronal reconstruction MIP image demonstrates that the left upper lobe pulmonary vein drains into the innominate vein (*arrows*). (**C**) The left upper lobe pulmonary vein is seen on this axial CT image (*arrow*) and could easily be mistaken for a left-sided superior vena cava.

◆ Total Anomalous Pulmonary Venous Return

- ◆ A cyanotic heart lesion with increased pulmonary blood flow presents in the neonatal period.
- ◆ The condition is characterized by a connection of the pulmonary veins from both lungs to form a confluence posterior to the left atrium and the connection of a venous channel from this confluence to a systemic vein, the right atrium, or both (**Fig. 2.17**). Blood passes to the left atrium via an atrial septal defect or patent foramen ovale.
- ◆ The connection is described as supracardiac (**Fig. 2.18**), cardiac, infracardiac, or mixed, depending on its location.

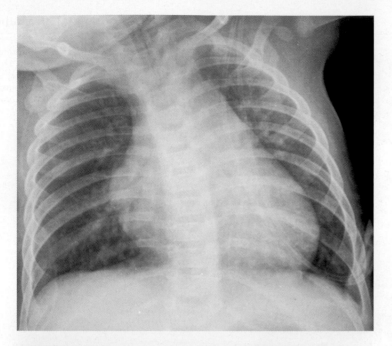

A

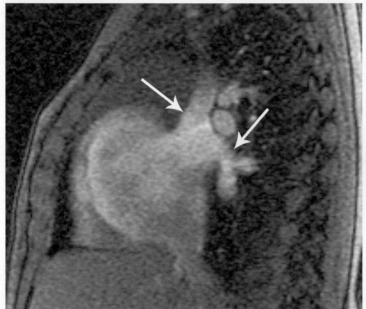

B

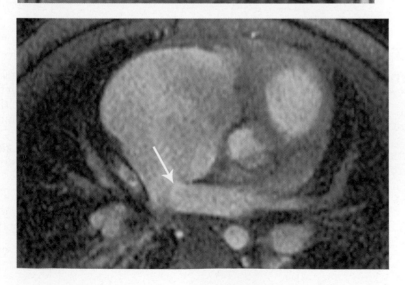

C

Fig. 2.17 (A–C) Total anomalous pulmonary venous connection in a 5-month-old boy. **(A)** The chest radiograph demonstrates some prominence of the right side of the heart. The pulmonary vasculature appears prominent. **(B)** Magnetic resonance image (MRI) demonstrates the right inferior pulmonary vein and superior vena cava (*arrows*) draining into a confluence before flowing into the right atrium. **(C)** Axial MRI demonstrates the left inferior pulmonary veins forming a common trunk before entering into the right atrium (*arrow*).

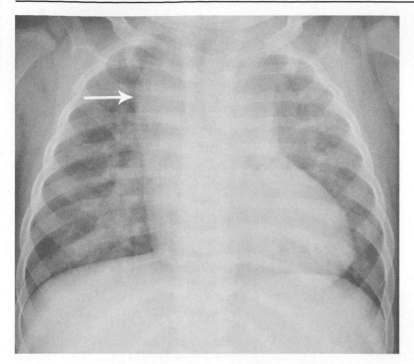

Fig. 2.18 Supracardiac total anomalous pulmonary venous connection in a 9-month-old boy. The heart is enlarged, and a dilated superior vena cava (*arrow*) and innominate vein result in the figure-of-eight appearance of the heart. An increase in the diameter of the pulmonary vessels (plethora) is also seen.

◆ The supracardiac and cardiac types are often not obstructive, but bilateral infracardiac connections are almost always obstructive because blood passes through the hepatic sinusoids.

Suggested Reading

Bush A. Congenital lung disease: a plea for clear thinking and clear nomenclature. Pediatr Pulmonol 2001;32(4):328–337

Castañer E, Gallardo X, Rimola J, et al. Congenital and acquired pulmonary artery anomalies in the adult: radiologic overview. Radiographics 2006;26(2):349–371

Do KH, Goo JM, Im JG, Kim KW, Chung JW, Park JH. Systemic arterial supply to the lungs in adults: spiral CT findings. Radiographics 2001;21(2):387–402

Goo HW, Park IS, Ko JK, et al. CT of congenital heart disease: normal anatomy and typical pathologic conditions. Radiographics 2003;23(Spec No):S147–S165

Uchiyama D, Fujimoto K, Uchida M, Koganemaru M, Urae T, Hayabuchi N. Bronchial arteriovenous malformation: MDCT angiography findings. AJR Am J Roentgenol 2007;188(5):W409–W411

Yamanaka A, Hirai T, Fujimoto T, Hase M, Noguchi M, Konishi F. Anomalous systemic arterial supply to normal basal segments of the left lower lobe. Ann Thorac Surg 1999;68(2):332–338

Zylak CJ, Eyler WR, Spizarny DL, Stone CH. Developmental lung anomalies in the adult: radiologic-pathologic correlation. Radiographics 2002;22(Spec No):S25–S43

3

Cardiac Disease

Heart diseases frequently cause pulmonary dysfunction because of the close structural and functional association of the heart and lungs. The pulmonary vasculature is normally a low-pressure, low-resistance system with high compliance and a large vascular reserve. However, in patients with a left-to-right shunt due to congenital heart disease, the elevations in pulmonary artery flow and pressure result in progressive pathologic changes in the pulmonary vasculature. This leads to an increase in pulmonary vascular resistance, irreversible pulmonary hypertension, right-sided heart failure, and reversal of shunt flow, a condition known as Eisenmenger syndrome. In this chapter, the effects of cardiac disease on the pulmonary vasculature are examined. Atrial septal defect, ventricular septal defect, and patent ductus arteriosus are used as examples of congenital heart diseases with a left-to-right shunt. The lung changes, as seen on imaging, of acute and chronic pulmonary venous hypertension are explained, and the pulmonary vascular changes seen in the acquired heart disease mitral stenosis are illustrated.

◆ Atrial Septal Defect

- ◆ Atrial septal defect accounts for one-third of cases of congenital heart disease detected in adults.
- ◆ Ostium secundum atrial septal defects, the most common type, are located within the oval fossa; ostium primum atrial septal defects are next in frequency, and sinus venosus defects are the least common.
- ◆ The sinus venosus defect is frequently associated with an abnormal connection of one or all of the right pulmonary veins.
- ◆ Echocardiography is the method of choice for the diagnosis of atrial septal defect.
- ◆ The chest radiograph characteristically shows dilatation of the central pulmonary arteries and an increase in diameter of the central and peripheral pulmonary vessels (**Fig. 3.1**).

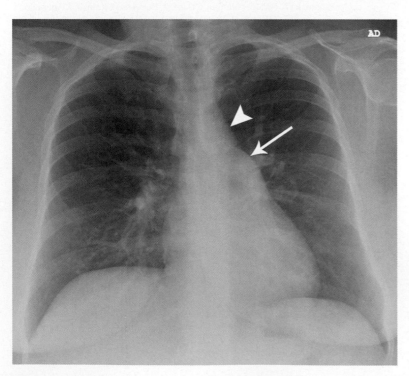

Fig. 3.1 Atrial septal defect in a 23-year-old woman. The heart size is normal; there is enlargement of the main pulmonary artery (*arrow*) and a small-appearing aortic arch (*arrowhead*). The pulmonary arteries centrally are mildly enlarged.

◆ Ventricular Septal Defect

- ◆ Ventricular septal defects are the most common congenital heart condition in infants and children.
- ◆ Of these defects, 70% are located in the membranous portion of the interventricular septum, 20% in the muscular portion of the septum, 5% just below the aortic valve, and 5% near the junction of the mitral and tricuspid valves with associated atrioventricular canal defects.
- ◆ Individuals with a large defect may progress to heart failure as babies (**Fig. 3.2**); those who survive until adulthood usually have pulmonary hypertension with subsequent right ventricular hypertrophy and dilatation.
- ◆ Ventricular septal defects are frequently associated with complex congenital heart disease.
- ◆ The chest radiograph may demonstrate a normal heart size or cardiomegaly. The pulmonary arteries show dilatation of the central vessels and an increase in diameter of the peripheral pulmonary vessels (**Fig. 3.3**).
- ◆ Cross-sectional imaging demonstrates the primary defect and associated defects (**Fig. 3.4**).

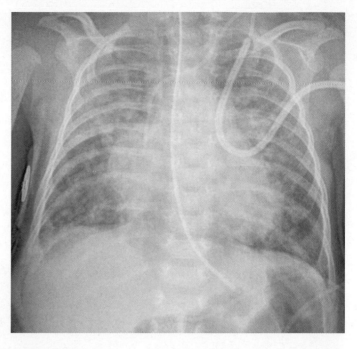

Fig. 3.2 Large ventricular septal defect in a 3-month-old boy. Chest radiograph shows cardiomegaly, prominent enlarged pulmonary vessels, and perihilar consolidation, consistent with alveolar pulmonary edema.

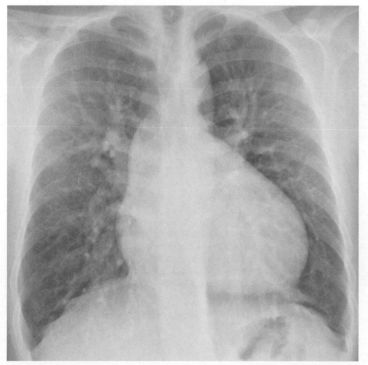

Fig. 3.3 Ventricular septal defect with infundibular stenosis of the right ventricular outflow tract in a 24-year-old man. The heart is enlarged. The pulmonary arteries centrally and peripherally are enlarged.

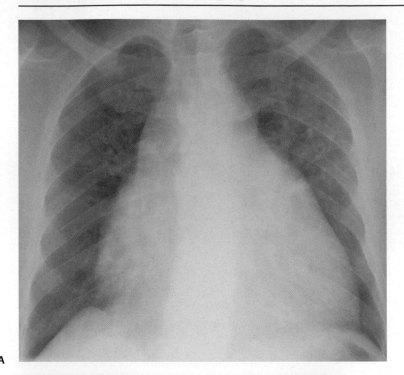

A

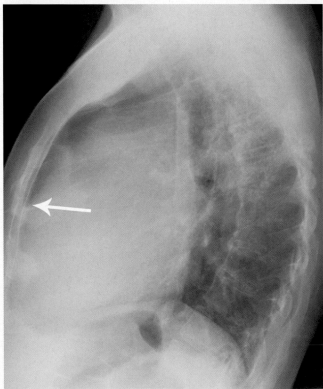

B

Fig. 3.4 (A–D) Ventricular septal defect in a 60-year-old man. **(A)** Chest radiograph shows that the heart is enlarged. The main, central, and peripheral pulmonary arteries are also enlarged. **(B)** Lateral radiograph shows dilatation of the right ventricle, evidenced by a decrease in the normal retrosternal translucency (*arrow*).

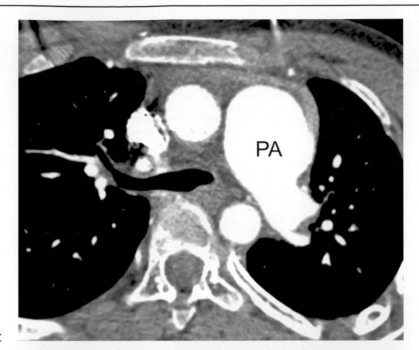

C

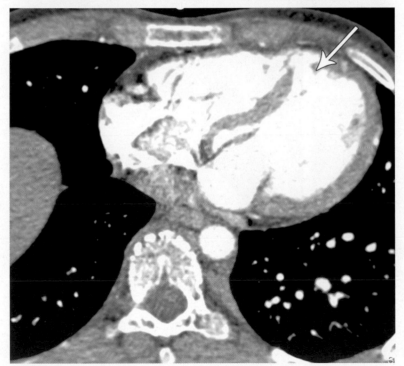

D

Fig. 3.4 (*Continued*) Ventricular septal defect in a 60-year-old man. **(C)** CT demonstrates a large main pulmonary artery (*PA*). **(D)** A CT image obtained further caudad shows the ventricular septal defect (*arrow*).

◆ Patent Ductus Arteriosus

◆ In the fetus, the ductus arteriosus connects the left pulmonary artery with the descending aorta just distal to the left subclavian artery.

◆ Post partum, if the ductus arteriosus does not close spontaneously, a continuous left-to-right shunt from the descending aorta to the pulmonary arteries occurs.

◆ Echocardiography usually is the diagnostic method of choice.

◆ Computed tomography (CT) plays a role in the evaluation of patent ductus arteriosus; it is used to assess the size and shape of the patent ductus arteriosus and to identify ductal calcifications before surgery (**Fig. 3.5**).

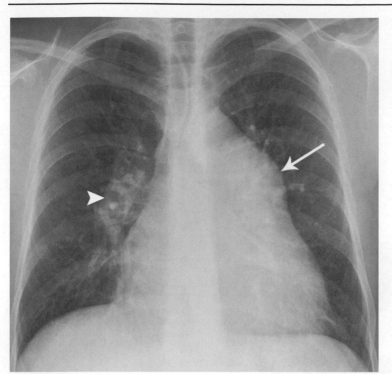

A

Fig. 3.5 (A–C) Patent ductus arteriosus in a 23-year-old man. **(A)** Chest radiograph demonstrates cardiomegaly with an enlarged left atrium and ventricle. There is a large main pulmonary artery (*arrow*), and the central pulmonary arteries are also enlarged (*arrowhead*); indicative of pulmonary artery hypertension. **(B)** CT demonstrates that the main pulmonary artery (*PA*) is massively dilated. **(C)** Maximum-intensity projection sagittal reconstruction CT shows the patent ductus arteriosus (*arrow*) between the superiorly located aorta and the inferiorly located, massively dilated pulmonary artery.

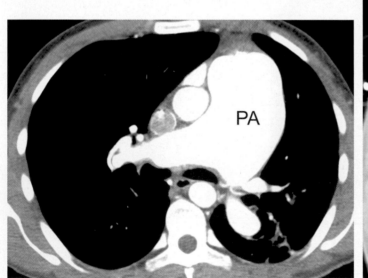

B

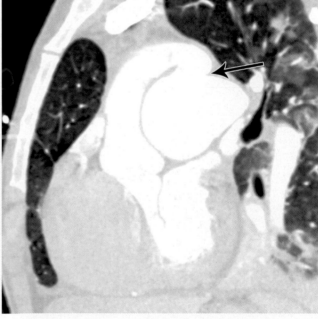

C

◆ Acute Pulmonary Venous Hypertension

◆ An acute increase in capillary hydrostatic pressure results in an increase in extravascular fluid in the lung, a condition known as interstitial and alveolar edema.

◆ A mean transmural arterial pressure of 15 to 25 mm Hg results in loss of definition of the pulmonary vessels, thickening of the peribronchovascular interstitium, interlobular septal thickening (Kerley lines), and pleural effusions (**Figs. 3.6, 3.7, 3.8, 3.9, 3.10,** and **3.11**).

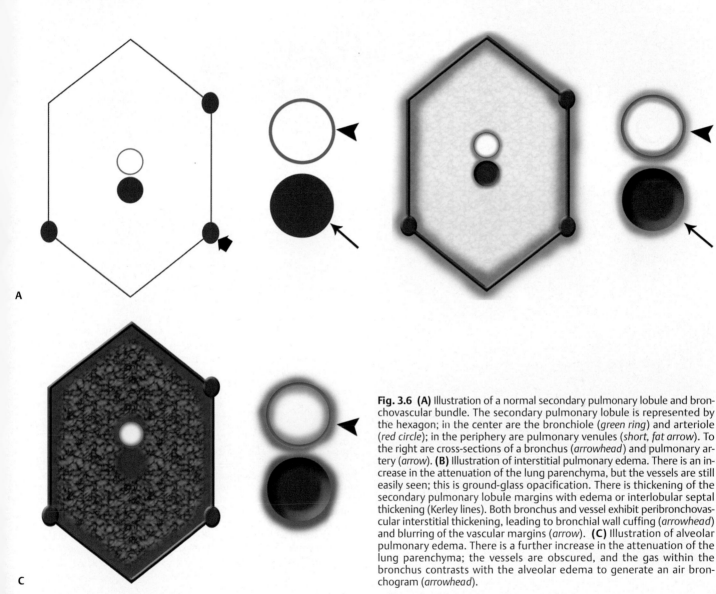

Fig. 3.6 (A) Illustration of a normal secondary pulmonary lobule and bronchovascular bundle. The secondary pulmonary lobule is represented by the hexagon; in the center are the bronchiole (*green ring*) and arteriole (*red circle*); in the periphery are pulmonary venules (*short, fat arrow*). To the right are cross-sections of a bronchus (*arrowhead*) and pulmonary artery (*arrow*). **(B)** Illustration of interstitial pulmonary edema. There is an increase in the attenuation of the lung parenchyma, but the vessels are still easily seen; this is ground-glass opacification. There is thickening of the secondary pulmonary lobule margins with edema or interlobular septal thickening (Kerley lines). Both bronchus and vessel exhibit peribronchovascular interstitial thickening, leading to bronchial wall cuffing (*arrowhead*) and blurring of the vascular margins (*arrow*). **(C)** Illustration of alveolar pulmonary edema. There is a further increase in the attenuation of the lung parenchyma; the vessels are obscured, and the gas within the bronchus contrasts with the alveolar edema to generate an air bronchogram (*arrowhead*).

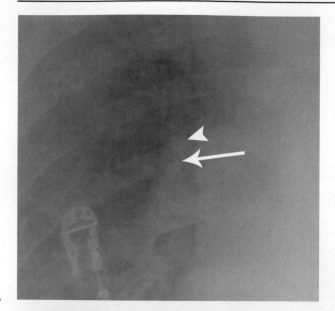

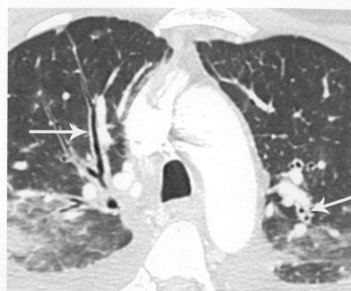

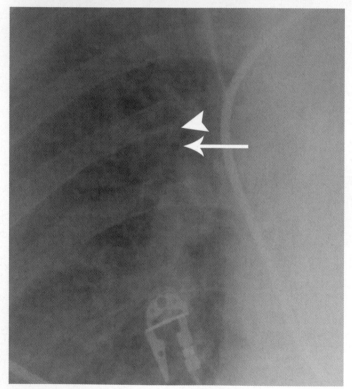

Fig. 3.7 (A–C) Interstitial edema in a 56-year-old man. **(A)** Peribronchovascular interstitial thickening is manifested on the chest radiograph as peribronchial cuffing of an end-on-right upper lobe anterior segment bronchus (*arrow*) and an increase in the apparent diameter of the accompanying artery (*arrowhead*). **(B)** CT demonstrates the same peribronchovascular interstitial thickening adjacent to the bronchi (*arrows*) and accompanying arteries. **(C)** Following therapy, in comparison with **A**, there has been a considerable decrease in the peribronchovascular interstitial thickening of the right upper lobe anterior segment bronchus (*arrow*) and artery (*arrowhead*).

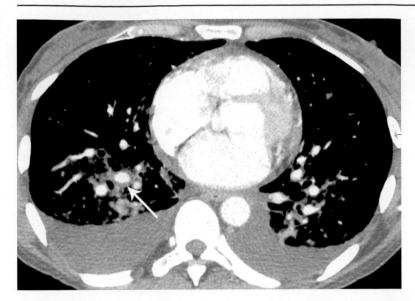

Fig. 3.8 Congestive cardiac failure in a 53-year-old woman. Contrast-enhanced CT demonstrates peribronchovascular interstitial thickening due to edema around a branch of the right inferior pulmonary vein (*arrow*) and adjacent bronchi and arteries. Bilateral pleural effusions are also present.

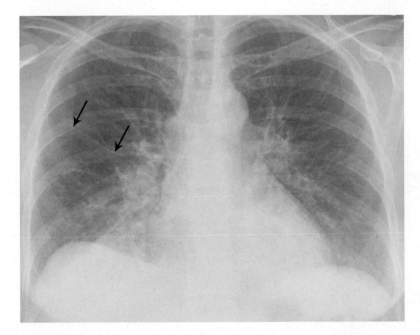

Fig. 3.9 Interstitial pulmonary edema in a 37-year-old woman. Chest radiograph demonstrates diffuse interstitial edema, some of which is manifested as long, thin lines radiating from the hila, also known as Kerley A lines (*arrows*).

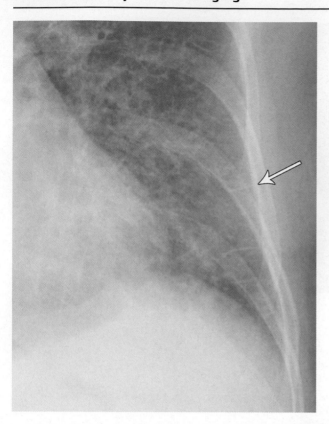

◆ A mean transmural arterial pressure above 25 mm Hg results in extension of edema into the alveolar spaces. This manifests as ill-defined acinar nodules, classically perihilar in distribution, that coalesce to result in frank consolidation (**Figs. 3.6C** and **3.12**).

◆ Acute mitral valve regurgitation secondary to papillary muscle rupture after myocardial infarction can produce right upper lobe pulmonary consolidation (**Fig. 3.13**). This radiographic pattern occurs because the plane of the mitral valve is inclined posterosuperiorly and to the right. The regurgitant jet is therefore directed preferentially up through the right superior pulmonary vein.

Fig. 3.10 Pulmonary edema in a 71-year-old man after acute myocardial infarction. Chest radiograph coned view of the left lower lobe demonstrates short, thin peripheral lines perpendicular to the pleural surface that extend to the periphery of the lung; these represent interlobular septal thickening or Kerley B lines (*arrow*).

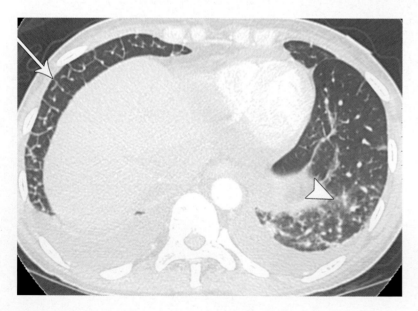

Fig. 3.11 Congestive cardiac failure in a 53-year-old woman. CT demonstrates smooth interlobular septal thickening (*arrow*), patchy ground-glass opacities (*arrowhead*), and bilateral pleural effusions.

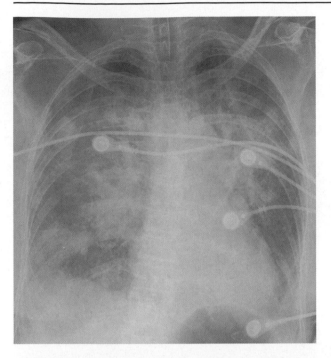

A

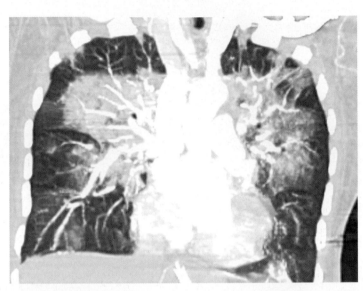

B

Fig. 3.12 (A,B) Acute pulmonary edema in a 57-year-old man in acute atrial fibrillation. **(A)** Chest radiograph demonstrates bilateral perihilar consolidation. Endotracheal tube, cardiac monitor leads, and bilateral pleural effusions are also seen. **(B)** Coronal reconstruction image of a CT pulmonary angiogram shows the classic "bat wing" distribution of alveolar pulmonary edema.

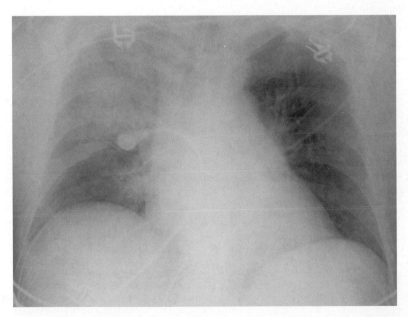

Fig. 3.13 Acute mitral valve regurgitation secondary to papillary muscle rupture after myocardial infarction in a 59-year-old man. Chest radiograph demonstrates the classic appearance of asymmetric pulmonary edema, predominantly affecting the right upper lobe.

◆ Chronic Pulmonary Venous Hypertension

- ◆ Mitral stenosis is a classic example.
- ◆ The first radiographic sign of chronic pulmonary venous hypertension is cephalization of the pulmonary vessels due to pulmonary vein and artery dilatation (**Fig. 3.14A,C**).

- ◆ Interstitial (**Fig. 3.14B**) and alveolar edema occurs at a slightly higher mean transmural arterial pressure than acute pulmonary venous hypertension because of an increase in vascular tone and remodeling.
- ◆ Lymphatic drainage is increased. This route of elimination of excess water takes time to develop and is not at full capacity in the acute setting. When the patient is in

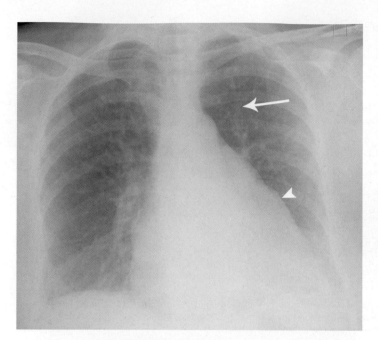

A

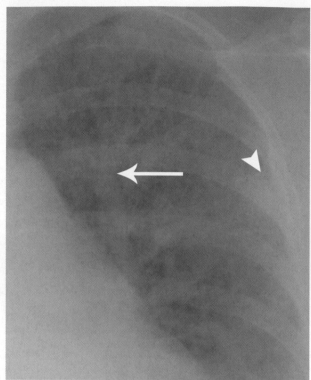

B

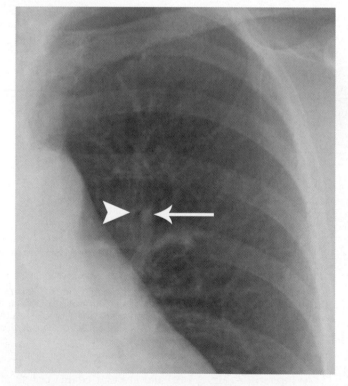

C

Fig. 3.14 (A–C) Mitral stenosis in a 43-year-old man. **(A)** Chest radiograph demonstrates cardiomegaly, an enlarged left atrial appendage (*arrowhead*), and upper lobe blood diversion (*arrow*). **(B)** Coned view of the left upper lobe when the patient was in heart failure demonstrates upper lobe blood diversion, blurring of the enlarged left upper lobe pulmonary vessel outlines (*arrow*), and Kerley B lines (*arrowhead*), indicative of interstitial edema. **(C)** Coned view of the left upper lobe after treatment demonstrates a normal-appearing end-on left upper lobe anterior segment bronchus (*arrowhead*) and a slightly enlarged accompanying artery (*arrow*).

heart failure, mediastinal lymphadenopathy is often also present (**Fig. 3.15**).

◆ Pulmonary venous hypertension can be one cause of pulmonary arterial hypertension. There is an increase in pulmonary artery tone as well as remodeling of the lung and vessels: alveolar fibrosis, thickening of the endothelial basement membrane, pulmonary artery intimal fibrosis, and medial wall hypertrophy. With early surgical correction, some of these changes can be reversed.

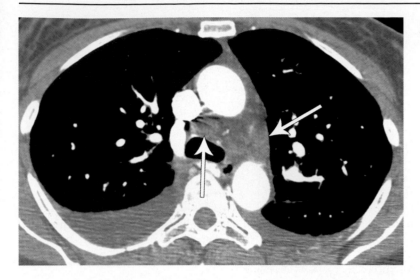

Fig. 3.15 An episode of heart failure in a 44-year-old woman. CT demonstrates enlarged lymph nodes in the left paratracheal and aortopulmonary window stations (*arrows*) and increased attenuation of the mediastinal fat.

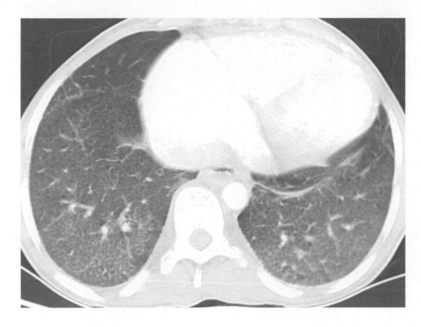

Fig. 3.16 A 27-year-old man with mitral stenosis and pulmonary hemosiderosis. CT demonstrates diffuse ground-glass opacifications and centrilobular nodules.

◆ Other lung manifestations of mitral stenosis include diffuse alveolar hemorrhage, pulmonary hemosiderosis (**Fig. 3.16**), and pulmonary ossifications.

Suggested Reading

Gehlbach BK, Geppert E. The pulmonary manifestations of left heart failure. Chest 2004;125(2):669–682

Gluecker T, Capasso P, Schnyder P, et al. Clinical and radiologic features of pulmonary edema. Radiographics 1999;19(6):1507–1531, discussion 1532–1533

Haramati LB, Glickstein JS, Issenberg HJ, Haramati N, Crooke GA. MR imaging and CT of vascular anomalies and connections in patients with congenital heart disease: significance in surgical planning. Radiographics 2002;22(2):337–347, discussion 348–349

Leschka S, Oechslin E, Husmann L, et al. Pre- and postoperative evaluation of congenital heart disease in children and adults with 64-section CT. Radiographics 2007;27(3):829–846

Remetz MS, Cleman MW, Cabin HS. Pulmonary and pleural complications of cardiac disease. Clin Chest Med 1989;10(4):545–592

Slanetz PJ, Truong M, Shepard JA, Trotman-Dickenson B, Drucker E, McLoud TC. Mediastinal lymphadenopathy and hazy mediastinal fat: new CT findings of congestive heart failure. AJR Am J Roentgenol 1998;171(5):1307–1309

Woolley K, Stark P. Pulmonary parenchymal manifestations of mitral valve disease. Radiographics 1999;19(4):965–972

4

Embolism

Acute thrombotic pulmonary embolism is the third most common acute cardiovascular disease after myocardial infarction and stroke and results in thousands of deaths each year because it often goes undetected. The prevalence of symptomatic acute thrombotic pulmonary embolism on dedicated computed tomographic pulmonary angiography (CTPA) is 12%, and the rate of coincidental pulmonary embolism on contrast material–enhanced CT is 1.8%. Diagnostic tests for thromboembolic disease include the following:

1. D-dimer assay, which has high sensitivity but poor specificity in this setting
2. CTPA, which is fast and accessible, with high sensitivity and specificity
3. Ventilation-perfusion scintigraphy, which has high sensitivity but poor specificity
4. Lower limb ultrasonography, which is a surrogate test with high specificity and rather low sensitivity
5. Pulmonary angiography, the "diagnostic standard of reference," which is underused
6. Magnetic resonance imaging (MRI), which has high sensitivity and specificity and is useful in cases in which iodinated contrast material and radiation must be avoided.

In this chapter, the diagnostic criteria for acute and chronic thrombotic pulmonary embolism on CTPA and angiography are illustrated, and the causes of the misdiagnosis of pulmonary embolism on CTPA are discussed. The imaging findings of acute thrombotic pulmonary embolism on ventilation-perfusion scintigraphy and MRI are demonstrated and the causes of nonthrombotic pulmonary arterial embolism illustrated.

◆ Direct Signs of Acute Thrombotic Pulmonary Embolism on Computed Tomography and Angiography

- Intraluminal filling defects that show a sharp interface with intravenous (I.V.) contrast material (**Fig. 4.1**).
- Complete arterial occlusion with failure to opacify the entire lumen; possible enlargement of the affected artery

in comparison with pulmonary arteries of the same order of branching (**Fig. 4.2**).
- A central arterial filling defect surrounded by I.V. contrast material (**Fig. 4.3**).
- A peripheral intraluminal filling defect that forms an acute angle with the arterial wall (**Fig. 4.4**).

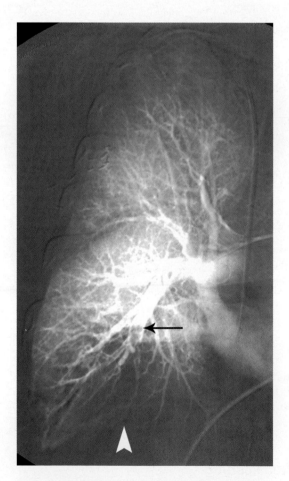

A

Fig. 4.1 (A–D) Acute pulmonary embolism in a 78-year-old woman. **(A)** Pulmonary angiogram of right pulmonary artery shows complete obstruction of right posterior basal segmental artery. Trailing edge or concave filling defect (*arrow*) is shown within column of contrast material. Perfusion defect within right posterior basal segment (*arrowhead*) is also detected.

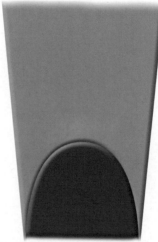

B

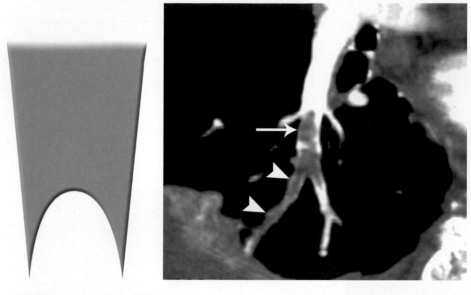

C

Fig. 4.1 (Continued) Acute pulmonary embolism in a 78-year-old woman. (B) Illustration of complete obstruction due to acute pulmonary embolism as seen on angiography. Trailing edge of thrombus forms concave filling defect within column of contrast material at level of obstruction. (C) Curved coronal reformatted CT image shows acute thrombus within right posterior basal segmental and branch vessels (arrow). More distal CT image is able to show expansion of the vessel with acute thrombus (arrowheads). (D) Illustration of complete obstruction due to acute pulmonary embolism as seen on CT. Both contrast material and thrombus are easily identified on CT, with acute thrombus forming acute angles with vessel wall.

D

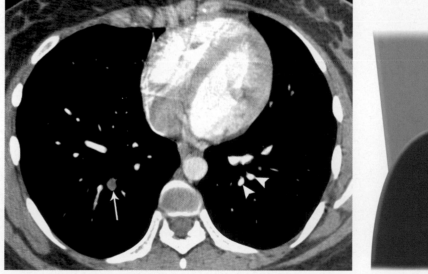

A

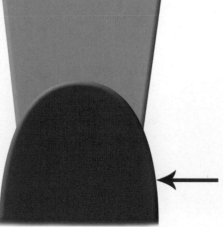

B

Fig. 4.2 (A,B) Acute pulmonary embolism in a 27-year-old woman. (A) CTPA shows thrombus (arrow) that expands diameter of right posterior basal subsegmental artery compared with pulmonary arteries of same order of branching (arrowheads). (B) Illustration of coronal reformatted CT image of acute pulmonary embolism shows expansion of diameter of involved vessel distal to point of obstruction (arrow).

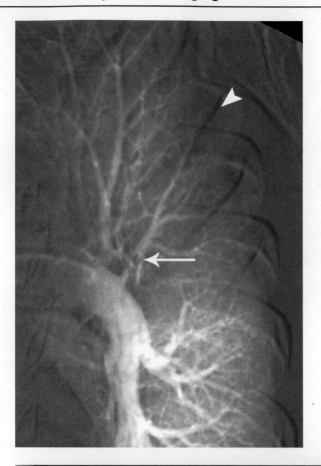

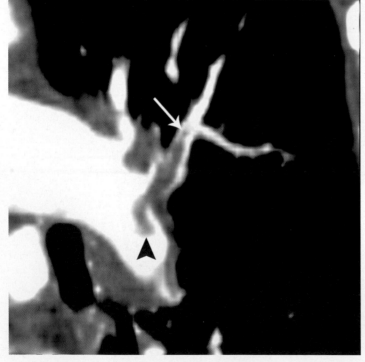

Fig. 4.3 (A–E) Acute pulmonary embolism in a 78-year-old woman (same patient shown in **Fig. 4.1**). **(A)** Left pulmonary angiogram shows central filling defect (*arrow*) within posterior segment of left upper lobe. In this patient, all three segmental arteries of left upper lobe arise directly from main pulmonary artery. Nonuniform arterial perfusion (*arrowhead*) is seen on arteriogram. **(B)** Curved coronal reformatted CT image shows nonobstructive filling defect (*arrow*). CT also shows more proximal nonobstructive thrombus (*arrowhead*) within main pulmonary artery, more easily seen on CT than on angiogram in **A**.

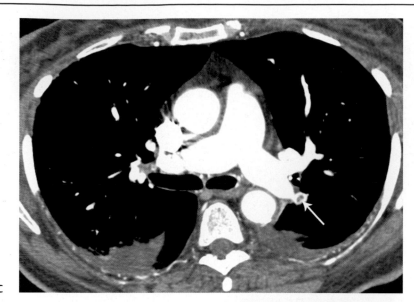

C

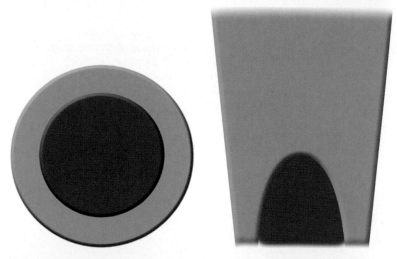

D

E

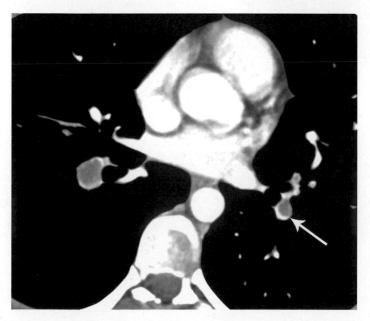

A

Fig. 4.3 (*Continued*) Acute pulmonary embolism in a 78-year-old woman (same patient shown in **Fig. 4.1**). **(C)** Axial CT image shows central filling defect within posterior segmental artery (*arrow*) of left upper lobe. **(D)** Illustration shows acute pulmonary embolism central filling defect on CT image viewed perpendicular to plane of thrombus; well-defined central thrombus is completely surrounded by contrast material. **(E)** Illustration shows acute pulmonary embolism central filling defect on CT image viewed in long axis of thrombus. Contrast material can be seen on either side of well-defined thrombus ("railroad track" sign.)

Fig. 4.4 (A–C) Acute pulmonary embolism in a 58-year-old woman. **(A)** CTPA shows thrombus within posterior basal segment of left lower lobe that forms acute angle with vessel wall (*arrow*). There are additional acute thromboemboli. (Continued on page 52)

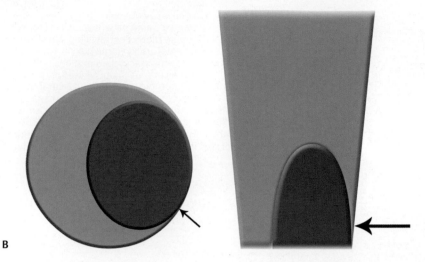

Fig. 4.4 (*Continued*) Acute pulmonary embolism in a 58-year-old woman. **(B)** Illustration shows eccentrically located filling defect on CT image viewed perpendicular to plane of thrombus; well-defined acute thrombus forms acute angles (*arrow*) with vessel wall. **(C)** Illustration shows eccentrically located acute thrombus forming acute angles with vessel wall (*arrow*).

◆ Indirect Signs of Acute Thrombotic Pulmonary Embolism

◆ Nonuniform arterial perfusion due to acute pulmonary embolism manifesting as a mosaic pattern of attenuation on CT (uncommon).

◆ Vasoconstriction distal to an obstructing acute embolism (Westermark sign) (**Fig. 4.5**).
◆ A peripheral wedge-shaped consolidation (Hampton hump) (**Fig. 4.6**).
◆ Pleural effusions.

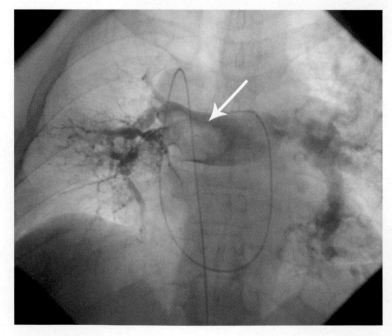

Fig. 4.5 (A–C) Acute pulmonary embolism in a 55-year-old man. **(A)** Right pulmonary artery angiogram shows large filling defect in right pulmonary artery (*arrow*). Nonuniform arterial perfusion is shown affecting most of right lung, with sparing of anterior segmental artery of right upper lobe. There is reflux of contrast material into left pulmonary artery. Unusual course of pulmonary artery catheter is due to azygos continuation of anomalous inferior vena cava.

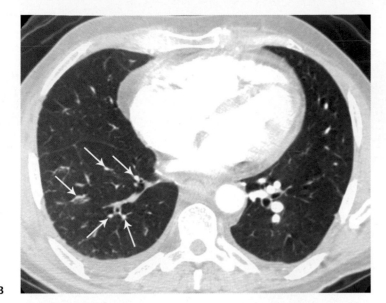

B

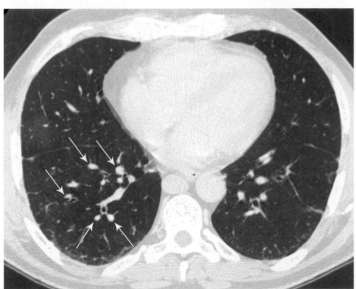

C

Fig. 4.5 (*Continued*) Acute pulmonary embolism in a 55-year-old man. **(B)** CT image obtained distal to large thrombus shows pulmonary arteries to have decreased diameter (*arrows*) with respect to adjacent bronchi and contralateral vessels. **(C)** Obtained 3 weeks after embolectomy, CT image shows pulmonary arteries (*arrows*) with normal diameter.

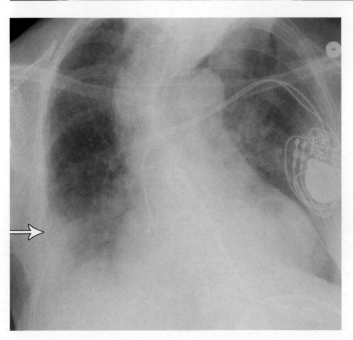

A

Fig. 4.6 (A,B) Peripheral pulmonary infarction in an 89-year-old man with acute pulmonary embolism of the middle lobe. **(A)** Chest radiograph demonstrates a peripheral wedge-shaped opacity (*arrow*). (*Continued on page 54*)

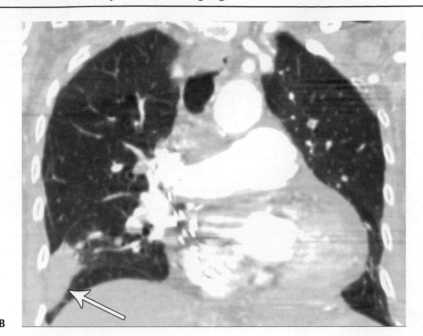

Fig. 4.6 (*Continued*) Peripheral pulmonary infarction in an 89-year-old man with acute pulmonary embolism of the middle lobe. **(B)** Coronal reconstruction CT shows correlative abnormality (*arrow*).

◆ Severity of Acute Thrombotic Pulmonary Embolism on Computed Tomography

- ◆ Right ventricular strain or failure is optimally monitored on echocardiography.
- ◆ Some morphologic abnormalities that indicate right ventricular failure can be quantified by CT. The most robust CT sign is right ventricular dilatation, in which the greatest right ventricular short-axis measurement is wider than the maximum left ventricular short-axis measurement (**Fig. 4.7**).
- ◆ The interventricular septum deviates toward the left ventricle.
- ◆ Reflux of contrast material into the hepatic veins indicates tricuspid valve regurgitation.
- ◆ A high clot burden score (>60%) is associated with a poor short-term outcome.

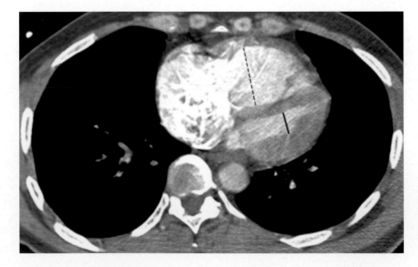

Fig. 4.7 Acute pulmonary embolism in a 42-year-old man who presented with chest pain and severe dyspnea. CT scan reveals that the short axis of the right ventricle (*dashed line*) is wider than that of the left ventricle (*solid line*), a situation caused by acute pulmonary embolism creating right ventricular strain.

◆ Direct Signs of Chronic Thrombotic Pulmonary Embolism on Computed Tomography and Angiography

- ◆ Complete occlusion of a vessel that is permanently smaller than pulmonary arteries of the same order of branching (**Fig. 4.8**).
- ◆ A peripheral, eccentrically located filling defect that forms an obtuse angle with the vessel wall (**Fig. 4.9**), which may calcify (**Fig. 4.10**).

- ◆ A band or web in a contrast-filled artery (**Fig. 4.11**).
- ◆ Flow of contrast material through apparently thick-walled arteries that are smaller as a consequence of recanalization (**Fig. 4.12**).
- ◆ Presence of an intraluminal filling defect with an acute pulmonary embolism morphology for more than 3 months.

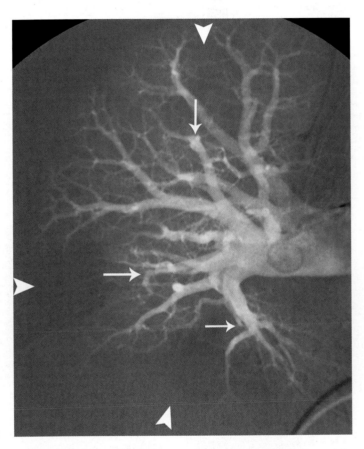

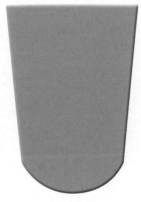

Fig. 4.8 (A–D) Chronic pulmonary embolism in a 40-year-old woman. **(A)** Angiogram shows complete obstruction (*arrows*) affecting subsegmental vessels of right upper lobe and lower lobe arteries. Resultant nonuniform arterial perfusion (*arrowheads*) is also well shown. **(B)** Illustration shows complete obstruction of vessel and convex margin with respect to contrast material. This is the "pouch" defect of chronic pulmonary embolism seen on angiography. (*Continued on page 56*)

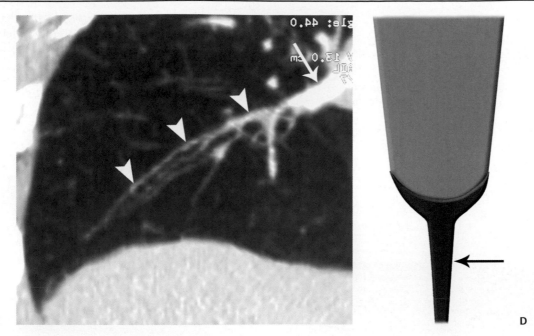

C

D

Fig. 4.8 (*Continued*) Chronic pulmonary embolism in a 40-year-old woman. **(C)** Curved coronal reformatted CT image viewed on lung window settings shows pouch defect of anterior basal segment of right lower lobe (*arrow*) with contracted distal artery, which is smaller than adjacent bronchus (*arrowheads*). **(D)** Illustration of reformatted CT image of complete obstruction in chronic pulmonary embolism shows contracted thrombus and artery (*arrow*) distal to pouch defect.

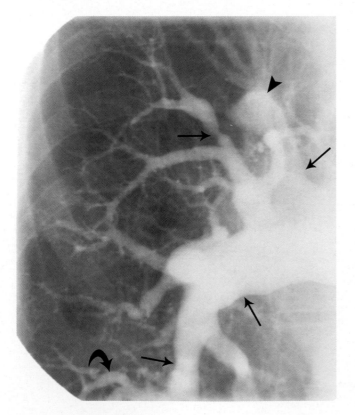

A

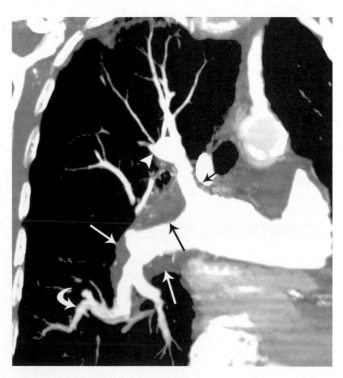

B

Fig. 4.9 (A–H) Chronic pulmonary embolism in a 60-year-old man. **(A)** Right pulmonary angiogram shows multiple intimal irregularities (*straight arrows*). Post-stenotic dilatation (*arrowhead*) is shown affecting posterior segment of right upper lobe. Also noted within right lower lobe is a tortuous vessel (*curved arrow*). **(B)** Coronal reformatted CT image shows organized thrombus (*arrows*) as cause of intimal irregularities. In addition, post-stenotic dilatation (*arrowhead*) is shown affecting posterior segment of right upper lobe. Also noted within right lower lobe is tortuous vessel (*curved arrow*).

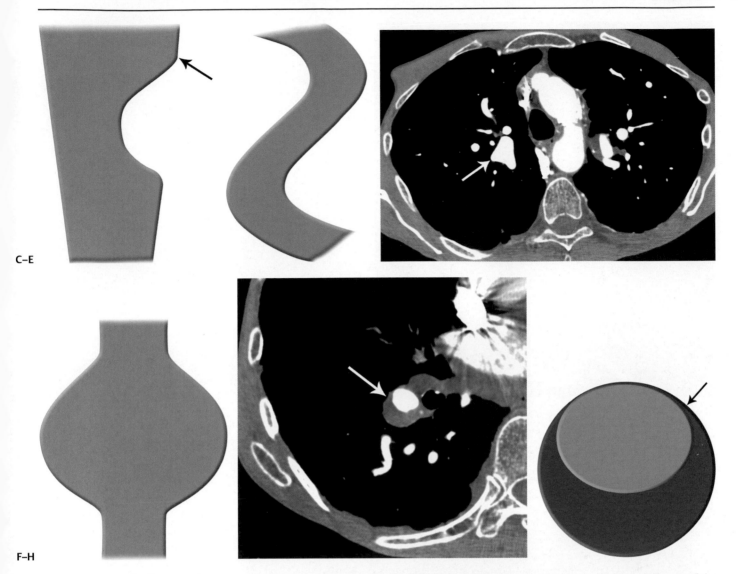

C–E

F–H

Fig. 4.9 (*Continued*) Chronic pulmonary embolism in a 60-year-old man. **(C)** Illustration of intimal irregularity of chronic pulmonary embolism as seen on angiography. This broad-based, smooth, margined abnormality can affect one or both sides of vessel; it forms obtuse angles with vessel wall (*arrow*). **(D)** Illustration of a tortuous vessel. **(E)** Axial CT image obtained at level of a pulmonary artery aneurysm shows that the posterior segment of right upper lobe (*arrow*) is affected. **(F)** Illustration of fusiform aneurysm with focal, concentric, symmetric widening of the vessel. **(G)** Axial CT image obtained at level of right lower lobe pulmonary artery shows eccentrically located chronic thrombus (*arrow*). Subcarinal lymphadenopathy is noted. **(H)** Illustration of intimal irregularity of chronic pulmonary embolism viewed in axial plane. This broad-based, smooth, margined, eccentrically located filling defect forms obtuse angles with vessel wall (*arrow*).

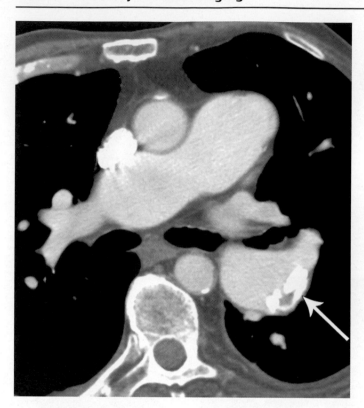

Fig. 4.10 Chronic pulmonary embolism in a 71-year-old man. CT demonstrates a heavily calcified thrombus that forms obtuse angles with vessel wall (*arrow*). The main pulmonary artery is also enlarged.

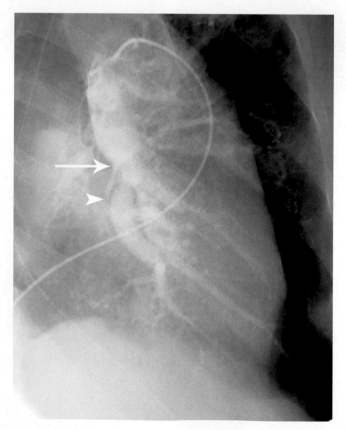

A

Fig. 4.11 (A–C) Chronic pulmonary embolism in a 51-year-old man. **(A)** Oblique view of left-sided pulmonary angiogram shows abrupt vessel narrowing (*arrow*) and complete obstruction of posterior basal segment of left lower lobe (*arrowhead*). It was difficult to see vascular band or web in this patient.

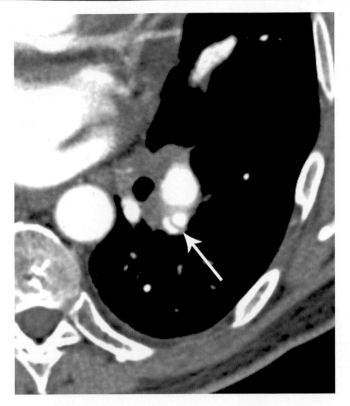

B

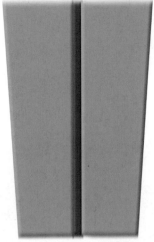

C

Fig. 4.11 (*Continued*) Chronic pulmonary embolism in a 51-year-old man. **(B)** Axial CT image obtained near origin of posterior basal segmental artery of left lower lobe shows band or web (*arrow*). **(C)** Illustration of nonobstructive filling defect of chronic pulmonary embolism. Band or web can be identified as thin, dark line surrounded by contrast material, often oriented in direction of blood flow.

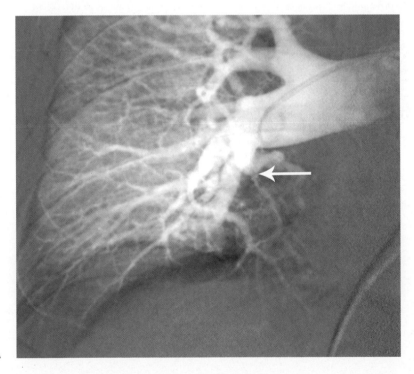

A

Fig. 4.12 (A–C) Chronic pulmonary embolism in a 65-year-old man. **(A)** Abrupt vessel narrowing (*arrow*) is shown affecting posterior basal subsegmental artery of right lower lobe. (*Continued on page 60*)

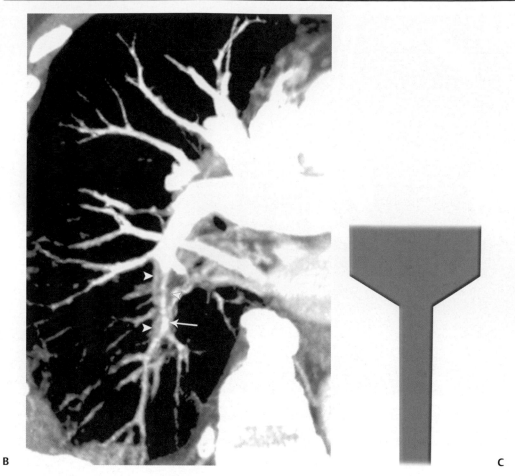

B

C

Fig. 4.12 (*Continued*) Chronic pulmonary embolism in a 65-year-old man. **(B)** Curved coronal reformatted CT image viewed on maximum intensity projection shows abrupt vessel narrowing that affects posterior basal segmental artery of right lower lobe. Note abrupt convergence of contrast material to thin column more distally (*arrow*). In addition, organized thrombus is identified surrounding column of contrast material (*arrowheads*). **(C)** Illustration of abrupt vessel narrowing of chronic pulmonary embolism as seen on angiography. This finding is recognized by abrupt convergence of contrast material to thin column.

◆ Indirect Signs of Chronic Thrombotic Pulmonary Embolism

- Nonuniform arterial perfusion due to chronic pulmonary embolism manifesting as a mosaic pattern of attenuation on CT (**Figs. 4.13** and **4.14**).
- Post-stenotic dilatation and aneurysm (**Fig.4.9A,B,E,F**).
- Tortuous pulmonary arteries (**Fig. 4.9A,B,D**).

- Enlargement of the main pulmonary artery (**Fig. 4.10**).
- Development of systemic artery–to–pulmonary artery anastomoses with enlargement of bronchial (**Fig. 4.15**), intercostal, and diaphragmatic arteries (**Fig. 4.16**).
- Hilar and mediastinal lymphadenopathy (**Fig. 4.9G**).
- Pericardial effusion.
- Pleural effusions.

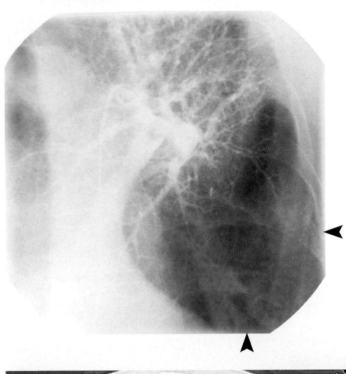

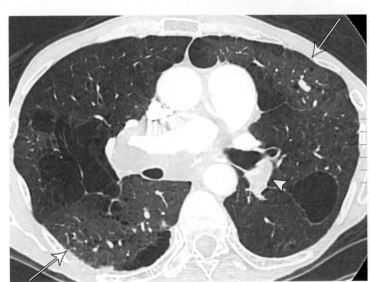

Fig. 4.13 (A,B) Chronic pulmonary embolism in a 60-year-old man. **(A)** Left-sided pulmonary angiogram shows complete occlusion of left lower lobe with nonuniform arterial perfusion and large perfusion defect affecting left lower lobe (*arrowheads*). **(B)** Axial CT image viewed on lung window settings shows occluded, contracted left lower lobe pulmonary artery (*arrowhead*). There is a decrease in attenuation of left lower and right upper lobes, and more normally perfused lung contributes to mosaic pattern of lung attenuation (*arrows*). Lung emphysema is noted incidentally.

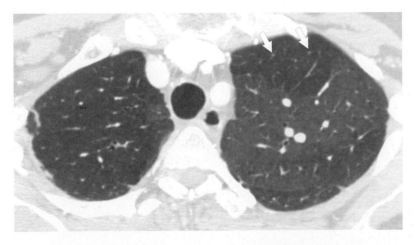

Fig. 4.14 Chronic pulmonary embolism in a 60-year-old woman with dyspnea. CT scan demonstrates a mosaic perfusion pattern. The dark regions of underperfused lung are seen to contain vessels (*arrows*) that are smaller than the adjacent patent vessels in the normally perfused lung.

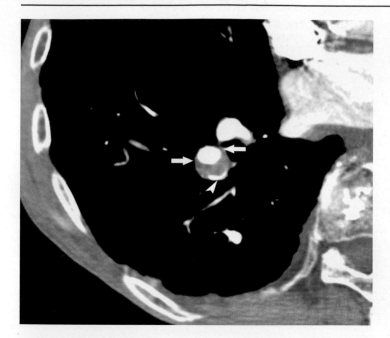

Fig. 4.15 Chronic pulmonary embolism in a 62-year-old man with dyspnea. CT scan shows an eccentrically located thrombus that forms obtuse angles with the vessel wall (*arrows*). Note the dilated collateral bronchial artery (*arrowhead*).

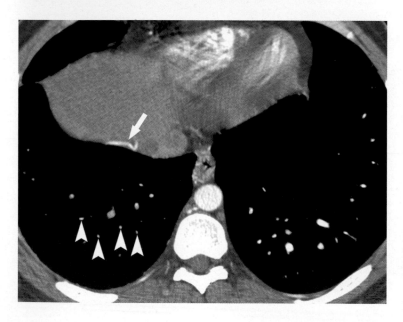

Fig. 4.16 Chronic pulmonary embolism in a 27-year-old man with dyspnea. CT scan shows complete occlusion of vessels in the right lung (*arrowheads*), which are smaller than normal vessels of a similar order of branching. Note the collateral blood supply from a branch of the right hemidiaphragmatic artery (*arrow*).

◆ Causes of Misdiagnosis of Pulmonary Embolism on Computed Tomography

Patient-Related Factors

- ◆ Respiratory motion artifact renders the diagnosis of pulmonary embolism at this anatomic level indeterminate (**Fig. 4.17**).
- ◆ Image noise due to increased quantum mottle is often seen in larger patients (**Fig. 4.18**).

- ◆ A pulmonary artery catheter for hemodynamic monitoring of critically ill patients can cause beam-hardening artifacts (**Fig. 4.19**).
- ◆ Bilateral lower lobe flow-related artifacts are due to transient interruption of contrast material enhancement as the consequence of a deep inspiratory effort just before CT scan acquisition (**Fig. 4.20**).

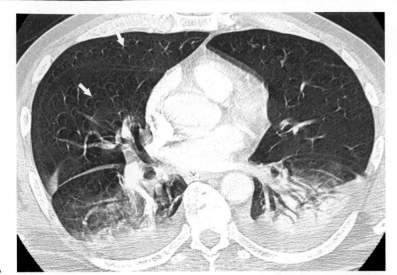

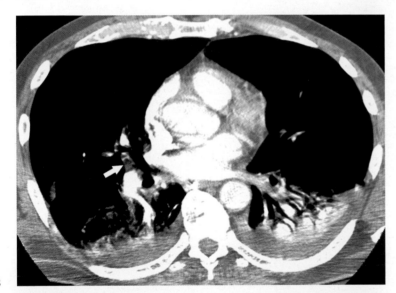

Fig. 4.17 (A,B) Respiratory motion artifact in a 61-year-old man with dyspnea. **(A)** CT scan (lung window) shows composite images of vessels ("seagull" sign; *arrows*). **(B)** CT scan (mediastinal window) demonstrates a low-attenuation abnormality caused by partial volume averaging of vessel and adjacent lung (*arrow*), a finding that can simulate pulmonary embolism.

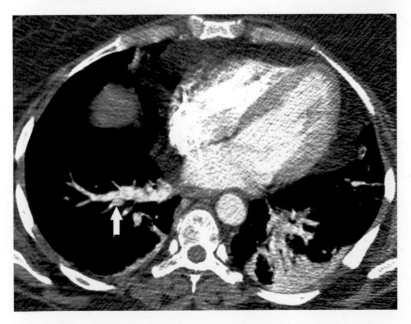

Fig. 4.18 Image noise in scans of a 39-year-old woman with chest pain. CT scan clearly depicts image noise pixels within the contrast material–filled heart chambers, a confluence of which could be misinterpreted as pulmonary embolism (*arrow*). Unlike true emboli, however, these apparent abnormalities are not well-defined filling defects. Small pulmonary emboli can be obscured by a large amount of image noise.

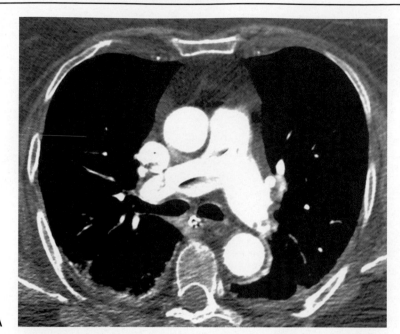

A

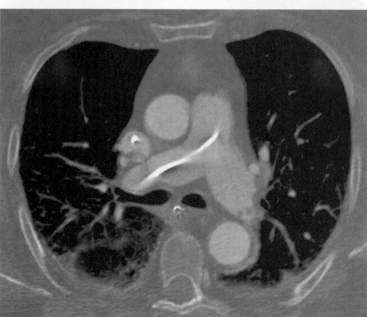

B

Fig. 4.19 (A,B) Beam-hardening artifact in a 63-year-old man with respiratory failure. **(A)** On CT scan, a pulmonary artery catheter causes adjacent beam-hardening artifacts within the main and right pulmonary arteries that mimic pulmonary embolism. Small pulmonary emboli are noted in the left pulmonary artery. **(B)** CT scan produced with bone window settings clearly depicts the pulmonary artery catheter. Adjacent beam-hardening artifacts are also seen.

Technical Factors

♦ Appropriate window settings are important to identify small emboli, webs, or bands (**Fig. 4.21**). A window width of 700 and level of 100 Hounsfield units (HU), or adjustment of the settings so that the heart valves are seen, can be used as an internal reference.

♦ Streak artifact from dense contrast material within the superior vena cava can obscure right pulmonary and upper lobe arteries. This can be reduced by using dual-chamber injectors to flush the superior vena cava with saline solution.

♦ The lung algorithm is a high-spatial-frequency reconstruction convolution kernel used to improve the quality of images of the pulmonary vessels, bronchi, and interstitium. This algorithm can create image artifacts that appear similar to pulmonary emboli (**Fig. 4.22**).

♦ Partial volume artifact is the result of imaging an axially oriented vessel with a slice thickness that is too wide (**Fig. 4.23**).

♦ Stair step artifact is the appearance of low-attenuation lines traversing a vessel on coronal and sagittal reformatted images and is accentuated by cardiac and respiratory motion (**Fig. 4.24**).

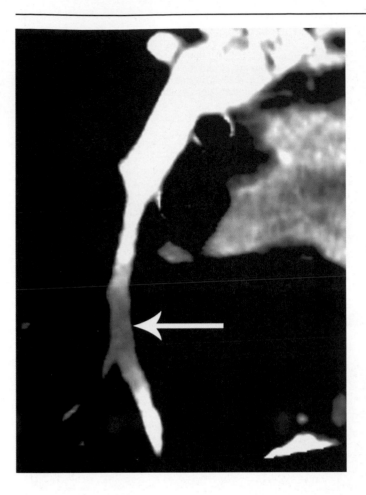

Fig. 4.20 Transient interruption of flow of contrast material in a 59-year-old woman. Coronal oblique reformatted image through right posterior basal segmental artery from CTPA shows segment of poor opacification (*arrow*) between areas of higher attenuation both proximally and distally. The interface between areas of low and high attenuation areas is ill-defined.

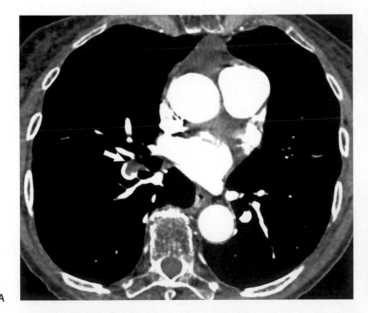

A

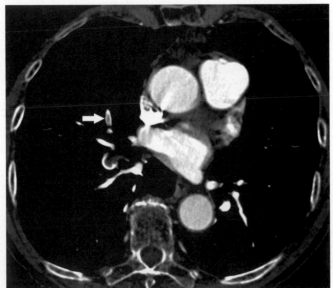

B

Fig. 4.21 (A–C) Acute pulmonary embolism in a 59-year-old man. **(A)** CT scan (window width, 400 HU; window level, 40 HU) demonstrates thrombus within the right lower lobe artery (*arrow*). **(B)** CT scan (window width, 552 HU; window level, 276 HU) shows acute pulmonary embolism within the medial segment of the middle lobe artery (*arrow*) that was missed on the image in **A**. The ideal window width is equal to the mean attenuation of the main pulmonary artery plus two standard deviations, and the window level equals one-half of this value. (*Continued on page 66*)

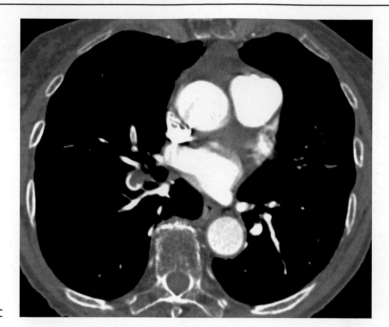

Fig. 4.21 (*Continued*) Acute pulmonary embolism in a 59-year-old man. **(C)** CT scan (window width, 700 HU; window level, 100 HU) demonstrates thrombus within the right interlobar artery and the medial segment of the middle lobe artery. **Fig. 4.21** illustrates the effect of different window settings on the detection of pulmonary embolism.

C

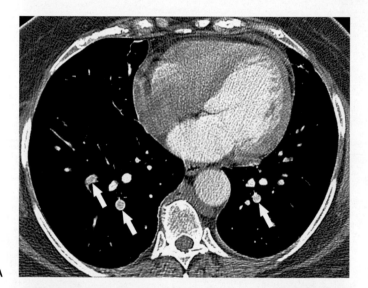

A

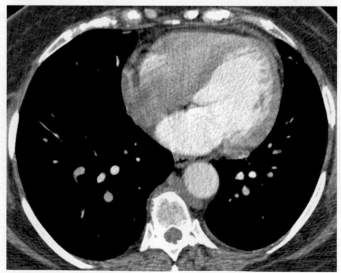

B

Fig. 4.22 (A,B) Lung algorithm artifact in a 70-year-old woman with dyspnea. **(A)** CT scan displayed with an edge-enhancing algorithm shows a lung algorithm artifact that mimics acute pulmonary embolism (*arrows*). This artifact occurs with mediastinal or pulmonary embolism–specific windows and manifests as a bright ring around pulmonary arteries, particularly if associated with a flow artifact. **(B)** CT scan displayed with the standard algorithm does not demonstrate this artifact; it does show less-than-optimal pulmonary artery opacification. No embolism was present.

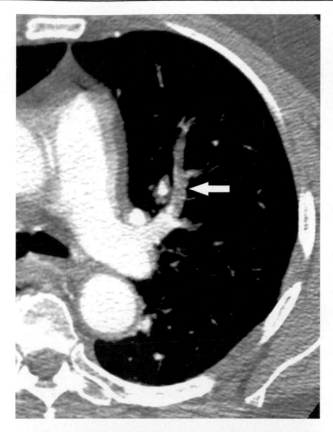

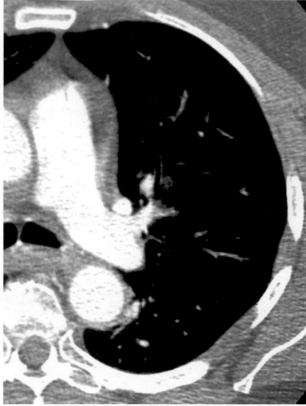

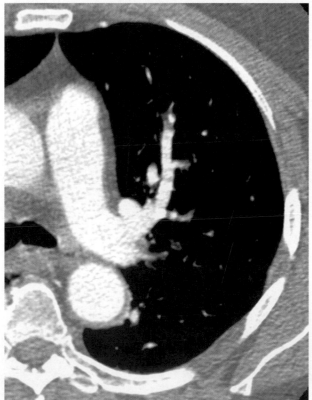

Fig. 4.23 (A–C) Partial volume artifact in a 52-year-old woman with dyspnea. **(A)** On a 3.75-mm-thick CT scan, partial volume averaging of vessel and lung creates an artifact (*arrow*) that mimics pulmonary embolism within the anterior segment of the left upper lobe. The apparent pulmonary embolism is ill-defined. **(B)** Contiguous CT scan obtained inferior to **A** demonstrates normal lung adjacent to the left upper lobe pulmonary artery. **(C)** Contiguous CT scan obtained immediately superior to **A** demonstrates a contrast material–filled pulmonary artery, a finding confirming that the low attenuation seen in **A** is due to partial volume artifact.

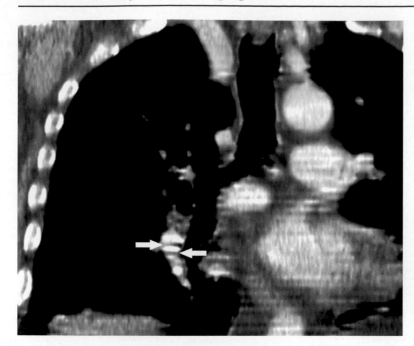

Fig. 4.24 Stair step artifact in an 84-year-old man with dyspnea and chest pain. CT scan shows low-attenuation lines that traverse a vessel on coronal reformatted images (*arrows*). This artifact can be recognized by its nonanatomic nature and is easily distinguished from pulmonary embolism.

Anatomic Factors

◆ Lymph nodes may be mistaken for pulmonary emboli. Knowledge of the hilar lymph node anatomy assists in differentiating lymph nodes from pulmonary embolism (**Fig. 4.25**). The use of sagittal and coronal reformatted images can help in difficult cases.

◆ Vascular bifurcations may simulate linear filling defects (**Fig. 4.26**). Sagittal and coronal reformatted images can help identify these normal anatomic structures.

◆ Unopacified pulmonary veins can mimic pulmonary emboli (**Fig. 4.27**). This pitfall can be avoided by observing veins to the level of the left atrium on contiguous images.

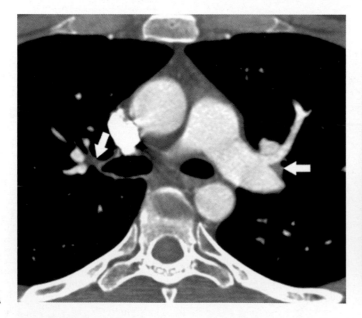

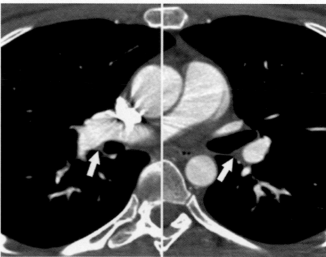

A

B

Fig. 4.25 (A–D) CT scans demonstrate normal hilar lymph nodes **(A)** in both upper lobes (*arrows*), **(B)** adjacent to the right and left interlobar arteries (*arrows*),

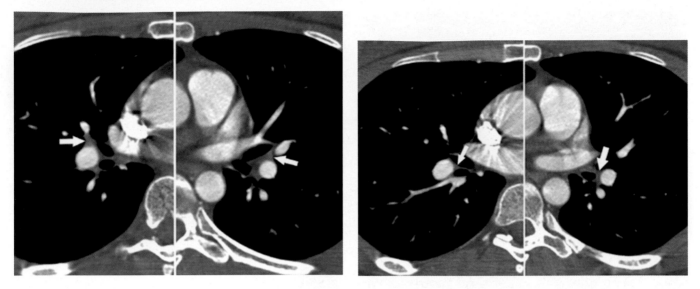

C

D

Fig. 4.25 (*Continued*) CT scans demonstrate normal hilar lymph nodes **(C)** in the middle lobe and lingula (*arrows*), and **(D)** in both lower lobes (*arrows*).

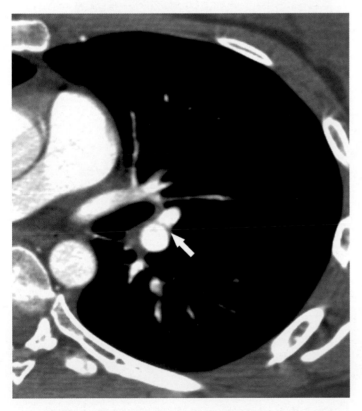

Fig. 4.26 CT scan shows the vascular bifurcation between the left lower lobe and lingular arteries as a curved line surrounded by contrast material (*arrow*). This could mimic a band or web of chronic pulmonary embolism. Contiguous images demonstrated the true nature of this finding.

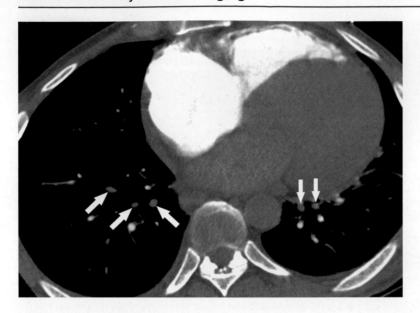

Fig. 4.27 CT scan shows unenhanced pulmonary veins (*arrows*), which can mimic complete occlusive pulmonary embolism. However, this pitfall can be recognized by observing veins on contiguous images to the level of the left atrium.

Pathologic Factors

♦ Mucous plug within a bronchus, which may also demonstrate peripheral wall enhancement related to inflammation, can mimic acute pulmonary embolism (**Fig. 4.28**).

♦ Perivascular edema can produce peribronchovascular interstitial thickening, which mimics chronic pulmonary embolism (**Fig. 4.29**).

♦ A localized increase in vascular resistance can result from lung consolidation or atelectasis; this can be a cause of an indeterminate CTPA (**Fig. 4.30**) and a misdiagnosis of pulmonary embolism.

♦ The Indeterminate Computed Tomographic Pulmonary Angiogram

♦ The major causes of indeterminate results are motion artifacts (**Fig. 4.17**) and poor contrast material enhancement. With faster scanners and attention to detail, these factors can be reduced.

♦ The minimum level of enhancement to detect all acute pulmonary emboli is 93 HU, and for chronic pulmonary emboli it is 211 HU. However, the results of a study may still be considered indeterminate because of the interplay of vessel size and image noise (**Fig. 4.18**).

♦ The radiologist should identify which images of pulmonary arteries are rendered indeterminate and whether additional imaging is necessary. For example, a study may be considered negative to the level of the segmental arteries and indeterminate at the level of the subsegmental arteries.

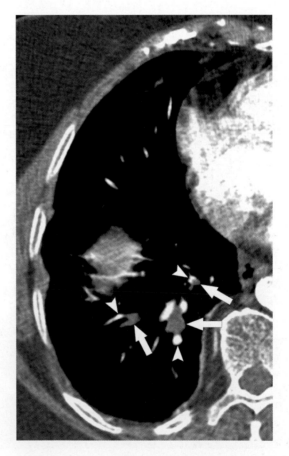

Fig. 4.28 Mucous plugs in an 83-year-old woman with dyspnea. CT scan shows mucous plugs (*arrows*), which can mimic acute pulmonary embolism. The posterobasal segment of the right lower lobe bronchus is dilated as well as filled with mucus. Identification of the normal accompanying pulmonary arteries (*arrowheads*) allows the correct interpretation of this finding.

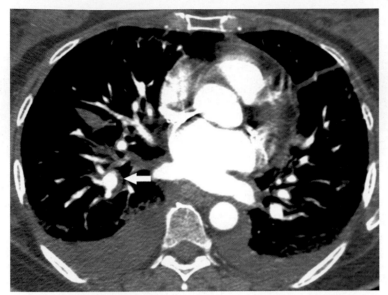

A

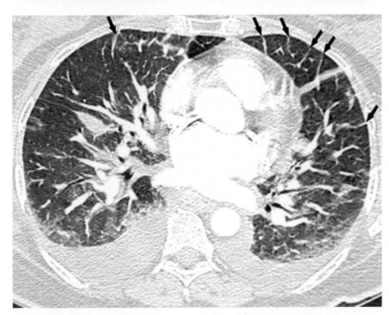

B

Fig. 4.29 (A,B) Left-sided heart failure in a 56-year-old woman with dyspnea. **(A)** CT scan shows peribronchovascular interstitial thickening caused by perivascular edema (*arrow*), a finding that can mimic chronic pulmonary embolism. **(B)** CT scan (lung window) demonstrates the accompanying findings of diffuse peribronchovascular thickening, ground-glass attenuation, smooth interlobular septal thickening (*arrows*), and bilateral pleural effusions. These findings indicate the true nature of the patient's condition.

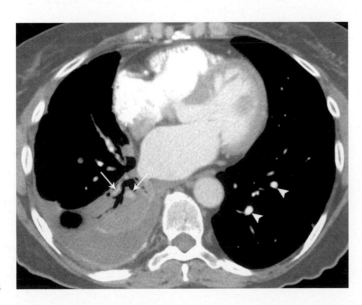

A

Fig. 4.30 (A,B) Localized increase in vascular resistance in a 69-year-old woman with breast cancer who has right-sided talc pleurodesis. **(A)** Staging CT was performed with injection of 65 mL of iopamidol (Isovue 370, Bristol-Myers Squibb, New York, NY) at a rate of 1.5 mL/s and a scanning delay of 35 seconds. Right lower lobe shows volume loss and consolidation. Note good opacification of left lower lobe pulmonary arteries (*arrowheads*). However, also note poor opacification of right lower lobe pulmonary arteries (*arrows*), indicating a localized increase in vascular resistance in right lower lobe arteries. (*Continued on page 72*)

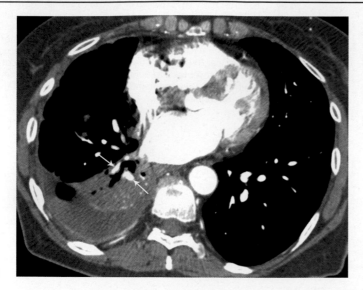

B

Fig. 4.30 (*Continued*) Localized increase in vascular resistance in a 69-year-old woman with breast cancer who has right-sided talc pleurodesis. **(B)** CT pulmonary angiogram 3 days after **A** with injection of 110 mL of iopamidol at a rate of 4 mL/s and a 22-second scanning delay. Note good opacification of right lower lobe pulmonary arteries (*arrows*). This image illustrates that peripheral vascular resistance can be overcome with the rapid injection of a large volume of contrast material and the acquisition of images at the very end of the injection.

◆ Interpretation of Ventilation and Perfusion Scintigraphy

- ◆ Ventilation and perfusion scintigraphy relies on the indirect signs of pulmonary embolism and the patient's chest radiograph is usually used to interpret results.
- ◆ The probability of pulmonary embolism with a normal perfusion scan (ventilation scan and chest radiograph may be abnormal) is 0 to 5%.
- ◆ A low-probability scan (10 to 15% probability of pulmonary embolism) is indicated by a single subsegmental perfusion defect (**Fig. 4.31**), any perfusion defect smaller than the corresponding abnormality on the chest radiograph, a nonsegmental perfusion abnormality, or matched ventilation-perfusion abnormalities (**Fig. 4.32**).
- ◆ An indeterminate (intermediate) probability scan (30 to 40% probability of pulmonary embolism) is one that indicates neither low nor high probability of pulmonary embolism.
- ◆ A high-probability scan (90 to 95% probability of pulmonary embolism) is indicated by two segmental mismatch defects (**Fig. 4.33**), one segmental and more than two subsegmental mismatch defects, or four subsegmental mismatch defects.

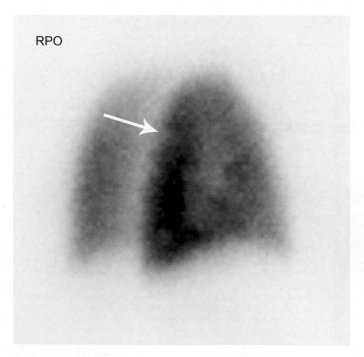

RPO

Fig. 4.31 Low-probability scan in a 37-year-old woman. Right posterior oblique (*RPO*) perfusion scan demonstrates a subsegmental defect in the right upper lobe (*arrow*). The ventilation scan was normal.

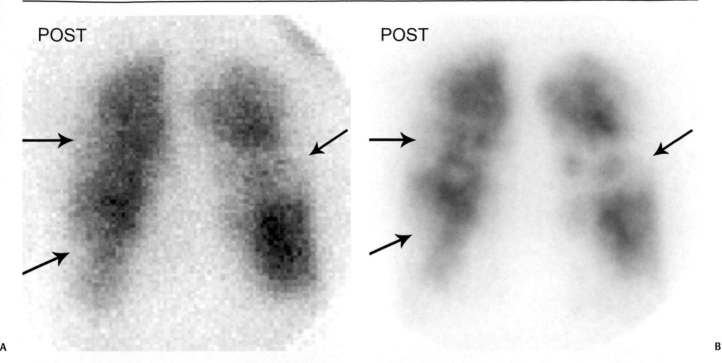

Fig. 4.32 (A,B) Matched defects in a 64-year-old man. **(A)** Posterior view (*POST*) ventilation scan demonstrates three ventilation defects (*arrows*). **(B)** Posterior view (*POST*) perfusion scan demonstrates three matched segmental perfusion defects (*arrows*).

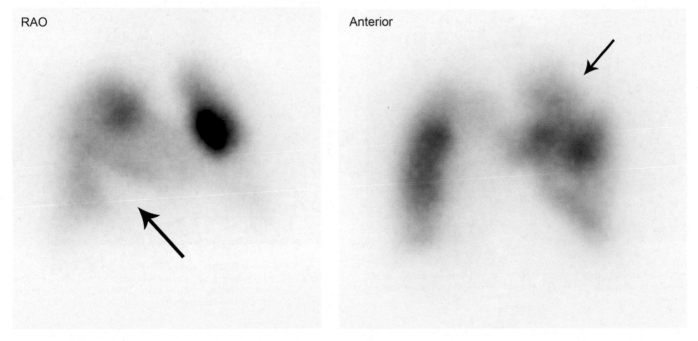

Fig. 4.33 (A,B) High-probability scan in a 58-year-old man with a normal ventilation scan. **(A)** Right anterior oblique (*RAO*) perfusion scan demonstrates a segmental defect in the right lower lobe (*arrow*).

(B) Anterior view shows a segmental defect in the left upper lobe (*arrow*), consistent with a high probability of pulmonary embolism.

◆ Magnetic Resonance Imaging of Pulmonary Embolism

- ◆ MRI has an inferior signal-to-noise ratio compared with CT and requires long examination and breath-hold times.
- ◆ MRI has the advantage of not using ionizing radiation or iodinated contrast material and can be an alternative to CT in selected patients.
- ◆ Vascular imaging with MRI can be performed with or without contrast material.
- ◆ Perfusion MRI can be used as a sensitive indirect sign of pulmonary embolism.
- ◆ The MRI diagnostic criteria for pulmonary embolism are the same as the CT criteria (**Fig. 4.34**).

◆ Coincidental Thrombotic Pulmonary Embolism

- ◆ Pulmonary embolism is seen on 1.8% of contrast material–enhanced CT scans and can occasionally be identified as a low-attenuation or high-attenuation filling defect on a non–contrast-enhanced CT of the chest (**Fig. 4.35**)
- ◆ Pulmonary embolism can be the cause of a high uptake of radiopharmaceutical on a technetium Tc 99m sestamibi (^{99m}Tc-sestamibi) scan performed for cardiac imaging and a fluorodeoxyglucose F 18 (^{18}F-FDG) positron emission tomography (PET) scan performed for tumor imaging (**Fig. 4.36**).
- ◆ Confirmatory imaging is recommended in these cases.

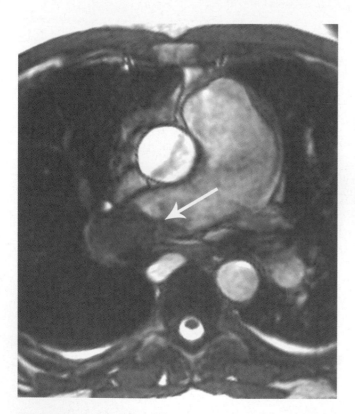

Fig. 4.34 Acute pulmonary embolism in a 27-year-old man. Contrast material–enhanced MRI demonstrates a well-defined filling defect consistent with a large thrombus within the right pulmonary artery (*arrow*).

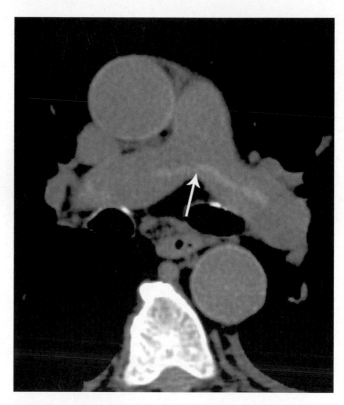

Fig. 4.35 Pulmonary embolism in a 67-year-old man with pancreatic neoplasia. The non–contrast-enhanced CT demonstrates a hyperdense saddle embolism (*arrow*) as well as embolism in the right pulmonary artery. This was confirmed on contrast material–enhanced CT.

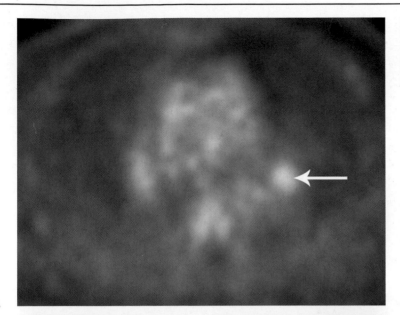

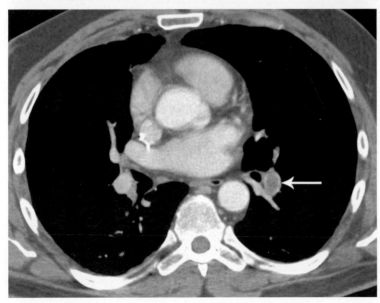

Fig. 4.36 (A,B) Coincidental pulmonary embolism in a 55-year-old man with a history of colon cancer. **(A)** ^{18}F-FDG PET scan shows focally increased uptake of FDG at site of acute pulmonary embolism (*arrow*). **(B)** Contrast material–enhanced CT scan shows acute pulmonary embolism in lobar artery of left lower lobe (*arrow*).

◆ Nonthrombotic Pulmonary Arterial Embolism

Air Embolism

- Iatrogenic causes of air embolism include injection of fluid including contrast material into venous catheters (**Fig. 4.37**), transthoracic needle biopsy, and barotrauma caused by positive-pressure ventilation.
- Air embolism is seen in up to 23% of patients given contrast material at CT. The risk for death is affected by both the amount introduced and the speed of introduction; the minimum lethal volume in humans is approximately 300 to 500 mL, and the minimum lethal injection rate is 100 mL/s.

- Clinical manifestations include sudden dyspnea, chest pain, hypotension, and convulsions.
- Scuba diving can be a cause of air embolism.

Catheter Embolism

- This iatrogenic cause of embolism is due to catheter tear, most often on catheter removal (**Fig. 4.38**).

Cement (Polymethylmethacrylate) Embolism

- The cement introduced during percutaneous vertebroplasty may cause pulmonary embolism via the external vertebral venous plexuses (**Fig. 4.39**).
- Symptoms are unusual.

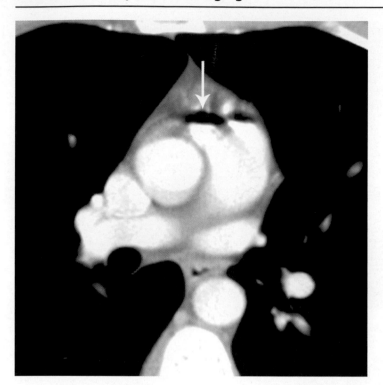

Fig. 4.37 Air embolism in a 34-year-old woman. CT demonstrates air embolism in the main pulmonary artery (*arrow*).

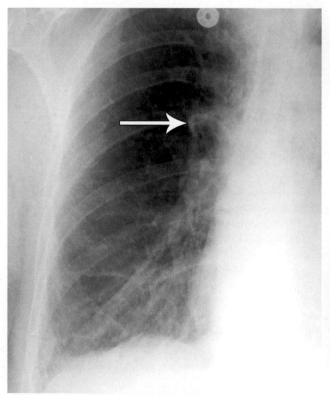

A

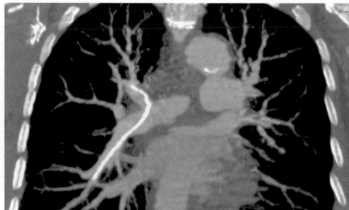

B

Fig. 4.38 (A–C) Catheter embolism in a 59-year-old woman. **(A)** Coned chest radiograph demonstrates catheter within anterior segment of right upper lobe pulmonary artery (*arrow*). **(B)** Coronal reconstruction CT shows the catheter in the right upper lobe, interlobar, and right lower lobe pulmonary arteries.

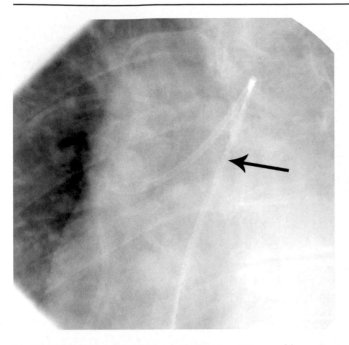

C

Fig. 4.38 (*Continued*) Catheter embolism in a 59-year-old woman. **(C)** Oblique spot view demonstrates a retrieval catheter (*arrow*) hooking around the catheter embolism.

Metallic Mercury Embolism

◆ Mercury pulmonary embolism is uncommon (**Fig. 4.40**).
◆ Most individuals who have received I.V. injections of mercury experience only minor toxic effects, although death has been reported.
◆ Symptoms can be attributed to infarction of the lung parenchyma.
◆ The prognosis is excellent.

Talc Embolism

◆ Talc granulomatosis is common among drug addicts who grind and inject intravenously medications that were originally intended for oral use only.
◆ The particles include microcrystalline cellulose, talc, and corn starch. These are trapped in the pulmonary vasculature, causing thrombosis, inflammation, and a giant cell reaction.
◆ Chest radiography and CT initially demonstrate small nodules and tree-in-bud opacities (**Fig. 4.41**). Eventually, large areas of increased opacification that resemble the progressive massive fibrosis of silicosis can be seen.

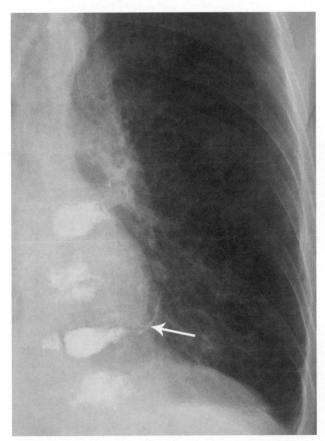

A

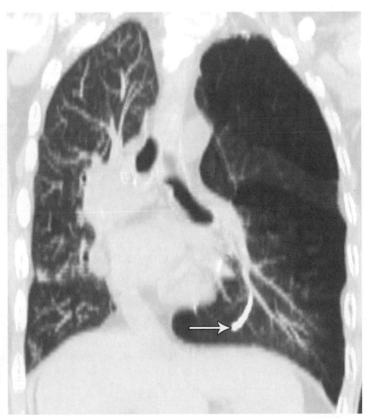

B

Fig. 4.39 (A,B) Cement embolism in an 83-year-old man. **(A)** Coned radiograph of the left lower lobe demonstrates multiple cement injections into the middle and lower thoracic vertebral bodies. In addition, there is a subsegmental cement embolism within the left lower lobe (*arrow*). **(B)** Coronal reconstruction CT on lung window settings demonstrates subsegmental cement embolism within the anteromedial basal artery of the left lower lobe (*arrow*).

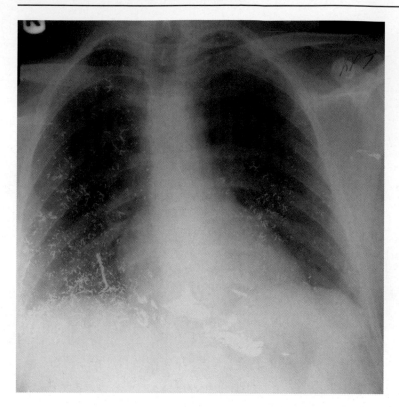

Fig. 4.40 Mercury embolism in a 23-year-old man resulting from self-injection. Chest radiograph demonstrates bilateral subsegmental branching emboli in the periphery of the lungs. Also of note is the presence of mercury in the left axillary vein, right atrium, and right ventricle.

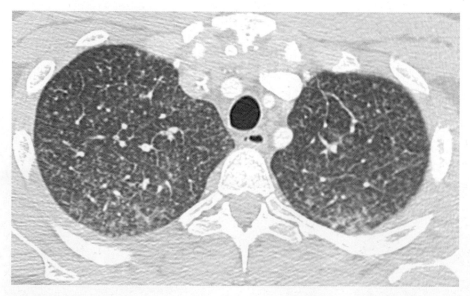

A

Fig. 4.41 (A,B) Talc embolism in a 27-year-old male I.V. drug abuser. **(A)** CT at the lung apices demonstrates centrilobular nodular and tree-in-bud opacities.

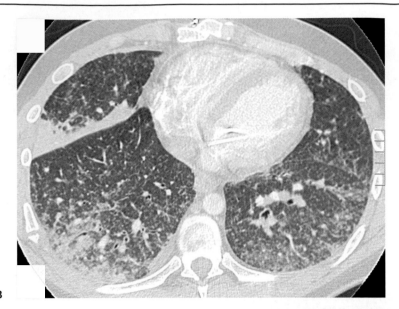

Fig. 4.41 (*Continued*) Talc embolism in a 27-year-old male I.V. drug abuser. **(B)** There are similar findings at the lung bases, as well as peripheral consolidation of the middle and both lower lobes.

B

Fat Embolism

◆ Fat embolism is an infrequent complication of long bone fracture but is relatively common after more severe trauma. Other causes include hemoglobinopathies, major burns, pancreatitis, overwhelming infection, tumors, blood transfusion, and liposuction.

◆ The production of free fatty acids initiates a toxic reaction and inflammation centered on the endothelium. Also, fat globules and aggregates of red blood cells and platelets cause mechanical obstruction of the pulmonary vasculature.

◆ The classic clinical triad of hypoxia, neurologic abnormalities, and a petechial rash occur within 12 to 24 hours after the traumatic event.

◆ Usually, 1 to 2 days elapse between the traumatic event and the appearance of radiographic abnormalities (**Fig. 4.42**); this allows differentiation from traumatic contusion.

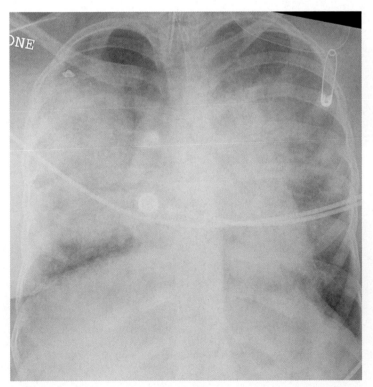

Fig. 4.42 Fat embolism in a 22-year-old man with acute fracture of the femur and pelvis. Chest radiograph demonstrates that the patient is intubated. The heart size is normal. Bilateral central and peripheral consolidations are noted.

Silicone Embolism

- ◆ Liquid silicone is used for cosmetic procedures by physicians as well as illegally by the general public.
- ◆ The "silicone syndrome" includes dyspnea, fever, cough, hemoptysis, chest pain, hypoxia, alveolar hemorrhage, and altered consciousness, which can lead to death in some cases.
- ◆ Similar to fat embolism, silicone embolism causes diffuse pulmonary hemorrhage and diffuse intravascular coagulation.
- ◆ The radiographic and CT manifestations resemble those of acute respiratory distress syndrome from any cause and consist of widespread homogeneous and heterogeneous areas of increased opacity (**Fig. 4.43**).

Amniotic Fluid Embolism

- ◆ Amniotic fluid embolism occurs in 1 in 9000 pregnancies, with an 80% maternal mortality rate in symptomatic patients. It can occur following cesarean section or normal delivery.
- ◆ It occurs when the embolization of amniotic fluid and fetal products to the pulmonary vasculature causes increased levels of endothelin-1, intense vasoconstriction, acute cor pulmonale, and circulatory collapse.
- ◆ Survivors of acute circulatory collapse have severe, diffuse intravascular coagulation.
- ◆ The radiographic findings resemble those of acute respiratory distress syndrome.

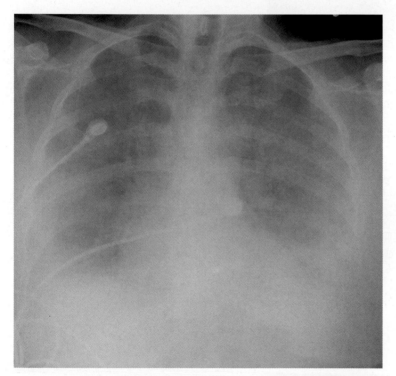

A

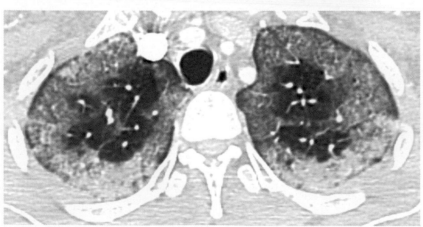

B

Fig. 4.43 (A–C) Silicone embolism in a 31-year-old man with dyspnea after buttock augmentation. **(A)** Chest radiograph demonstrates diffuse ground-glass opacification and bilateral peripheral consolidation. **(B)** High-resolution CT of the lung apices demonstrates peripheral ground-glass opacities with denser centrilobular and tree-in-bud opacities, as well as posterior consolidation.

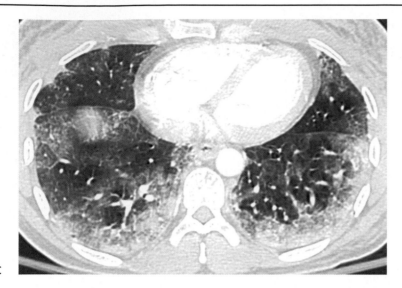

C

Fig. 4.43 (*Continued*) Silicone embolism in a 31-year-old man with dyspnea after buttock augmentation. **(C)** The lung bases demonstrate peripheral ground-glass opacities with denser centrilobular and tree-in-bud opacities, as well as some interlobular septal thickening and posterior consolidation. (Courtesy of Dr. Carlos S. Restrepo.)

Tumor Embolism

◆ Multifocal micrometastatic tumor embolism that is associated with dyspnea most often occurs in patients with carcinomas of the breast, lung, stomach, or prostate gland.

◆ Tumor emboli that affect subsegmental arteries can produce vascular dilatation and beading that, without treatment, increase in size over time.

◆ Small tumor emboli can affect secondary pulmonary lobule arterioles and have a centrilobular nodule or tree-in-bud appearance (**Fig. 4.44**).

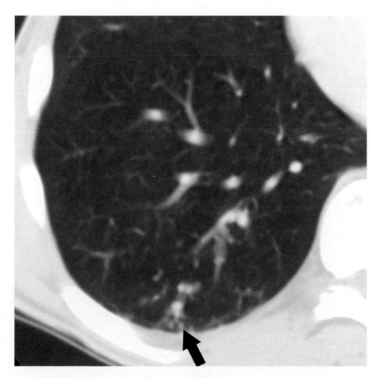

Fig. 4.44 Tumor embolism in a 60-year-old man with dyspnea and primary renal cell carcinoma. CT scan shows tumor emboli with a tree-in-bud appearance within secondary pulmonary lobule arterioles (*arrow*).

Suggested Reading

Han D, Lee KS, Franquet T, et al. Thrombotic and nonthrombotic pulmonary arterial embolism: spectrum of imaging findings. Radiographics 2003; 23(6):1521–1539

Hui GC, Legasto A, Wittram C. The prevalence of symptomatic and coincidental pulmonary embolism on computed tomography. J Comput Assist Tomogr 2008;32(5):783–787

Jones SE, Wittram C. The indeterminate CT pulmonary angiogram: imaging characteristics and patient clinical outcome. Radiology 2005;237(1): 329–337

Kluge A, Luboldt W, Bachmann G. Acute pulmonary embolism to the subsegmental level: diagnostic accuracy of three MRI techniques compared with 16-MDCT. AJR Am J Roentgenol 2006;187(1):W7–W14

Schmid A, Tzur A, Leshko L, Krieger BP. Silicone embolism syndrome: a case report, review of the literature, and comparison with fat embolism syndrome. Chest 2005;127(6):2276–2281

Stein PD, Fowler SE, Goodman LR, et al; PIOPED II Investigators. Multidetector computed tomography for acute pulmonary embolism. N Engl J Med 2006;354(22):2317–2327

The PIOPED Investigators. Value of the ventilation/perfusion scan in acute pulmonary embolism. Results of the prospective investigation of pulmonary embolism diagnosis (PIOPED). JAMA 1990;263(20):2753–2759

van der Meer RW, Pattynama PM, van Strijen MJ, et al. Right ventricular dysfunction and pulmonary obstruction index at helical CT: prediction of clinical outcome during 3-month follow-up in patients with acute pulmonary embolism. Radiology 2005;235(3):798–803

Wittram C. How I do it: CT pulmonary angiography. AJR Am J Roentgenol 2007;188(5):1255–1261

Wittram C, Jones SE, Scott JA. 99mTc sestamibi uptake by acute pulmonary embolism. AJR Am J Roentgenol 2006;187(6):1611–1613

Wittram C, Kalra MK, Maher MM, Greenfield A, McLoud TC, Shepard JA. Acute and chronic pulmonary emboli: angiography-CT correlation. AJR Am J Roentgenol 2006;186(6 Suppl 2)S421–S429

Wittram C, Maher MM, Halpern EF, Shepard JA. Attenuation of acute and chronic pulmonary emboli. Radiology 2005;235(3):1050–1054

Wittram C, Maher MM, Yoo AJ, Kalra MK, Shepard JA, McLoud TC. CT angiography of pulmonary embolism: diagnostic criteria and causes of misdiagnosis. Radiographics 2004;24(5):1219–1238

Wittram C, Scott JA. 18F-FDG PET of pulmonary embolism. AJR Am J Roentgenol 2007;189(1):171–176

Wittram C, Waltman AC, Shepard JA, Halpern E, Goodman LR. Discordance between CT and angiography in the PIOPED II study. Radiology 2007;244(3):883–889

Wittram C, Yoo AJ. Transient interruption of contrast on CT pulmonary angiography: proof of mechanism. J Thorac Imaging 2007;22(2): 125–129

5

In Situ Thrombosis

In 1860, Virchow postulated that thrombus can form as a result of vessel injury, disturbance of blood flow and hypercoagulability. A spectrum of diseases can be associated with one or all three of these precipitating factors, with the aftereffect of in situ thrombosis in the pulmonary vasculature. The criteria for in situ thrombus include (1) the presence of thrombus at the site of vessel injury and/or site of disturbance of blood flow and (2) the absence of other pulmonary vessel thrombi remote from the site of vessel abnormality. This chapter illustrates examples of in situ thrombosis of the pulmonary arteries and veins.

◆ Tumor-Related Pulmonary Artery Thrombosis

- In patients who have lung cancer, all three factors may be present: vessel injury from local tumor invasion, disturbance of blood flow, and hypercoagulability (**Fig. 5.1**).
- The differentiation between direct tumor growth along a vessel lumen and in situ thrombosis may be impossible based on imaging at one time point. Pathologically, the two often coexist.

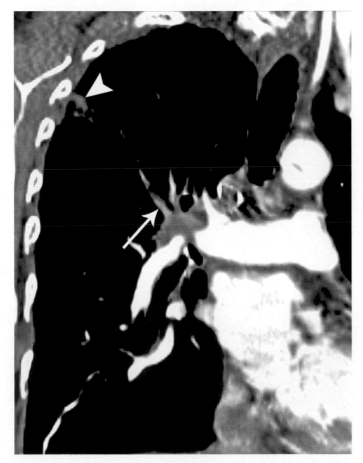

A

Fig. 5.1 (A,B) Peripheral infarction in a 71-year-old man with central adenocarcinoma of the lung. **(A)** Coronal reconstruction CT demonstrates the primary lung neoplasm invading the right pulmonary artery and a filling defect within the posterior segmental artery of the right upper lobe (*arrow*). There is also a peripheral pulmonary opacity (*arrowhead*). (*Continued on page 84*)

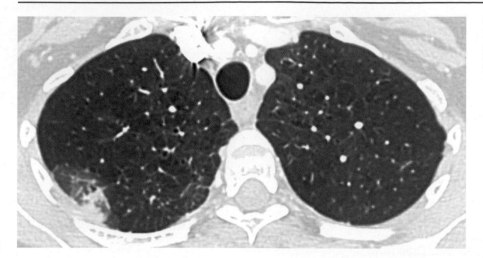

Fig. 5.1 (*Continued*) Peripheral infarction in a 71-year-old man with central adenocarcinoma of the lung. **(B)** On axial CT, this opacity has almost a wedge-shaped configuration, consistent with peripheral infarction.

B

◆ Radiotherapy-Related Pulmonary Artery Thrombosis

- ◆ The early effects of radiation on endothelial cells are characterized by swelling and sloughing.
- ◆ Such vessel-wall injury can lead to in situ thrombosis (**Fig. 5.2**).

◆ Pulmonary Artery Stump Thrombosis

- ◆ In patients who have undergone resection for lung cancer, all three prothrombotic factors are present: vessel injury, disturbance of blood flow, and hypercoagulability.
- ◆ The prevalence is 12%.
- ◆ There is a relationship between stump length and the development of in situ thrombosis.
- ◆ The shape of the thrombus can be convex (**Fig. 5.3**) or concave (**Fig. 5.4**).
- ◆ Stump thrombosis appears to have a benign natural history.

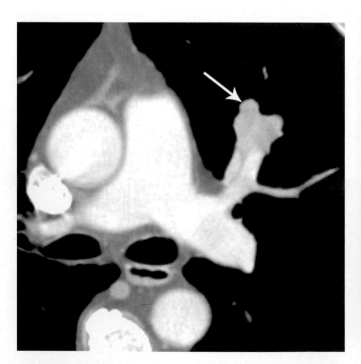

A

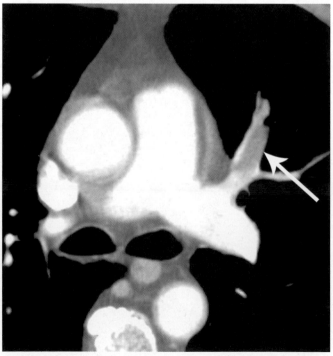

B

Fig. 5.2 (A,B) Primary squamous cell carcinoma of the lung in a 74-year-old man. **(A)** CT demonstrates the tumor immediately adjacent to the anterior segmental artery of the left upper lobe (*arrow*). **(B)** After radiotherapy, there is now a well-defined filling defect within the anterior segmental artery of the left upper lobe, consistent with in situ thrombosis (*arrow*).

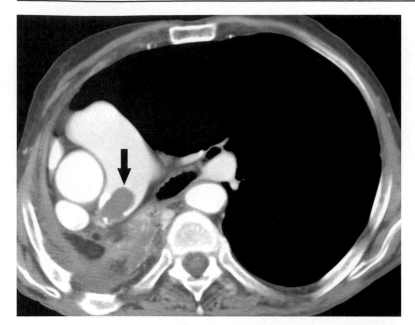

Fig. 5.3 Pulmonary artery stump in situ thrombosis in a 69-year-old man who underwent right pneumonectomy for lung cancer. CT scan demonstrates a convex pulmonary artery stump in situ thrombosis affecting the right pulmonary artery (*arrow*).

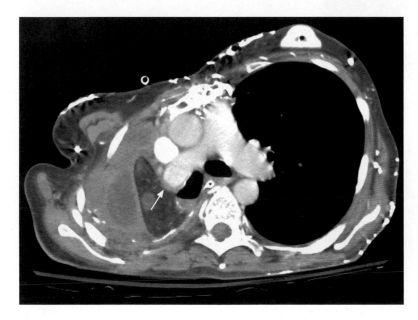

Fig. 5.4 Pulmonary artery stump thrombosis in a 55-year-old woman who underwent right pneumonectomy for recurrent chest infection resulting from post-irradiation fibrosis. CT scan at the level of main pulmonary artery obtained 9 months after pneumonectomy shows intravascular soft tissue that has a concave margin with respect to the contrast material (*arrow*).

◆ Infection-Related Pulmonary Artery Thrombosis

◆ Localized vessel inflammation from lung infection leads to an increase in the production of tissue factor and the inhibition of fibrinolysis.

◆ In this procoagulant environment, focal in situ thrombosis can occur (**Fig. 5.5**).
◆ Overt disseminated intravascular coagulation is seen in a minority of patients.

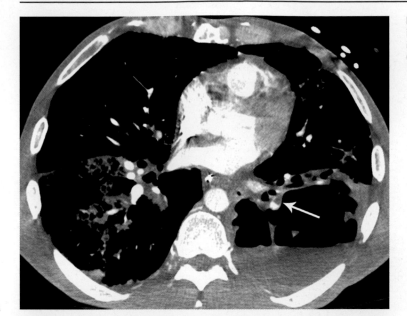

Fig. 5.5 (A,B) Staphylococcal abscess and in situ thrombosis in a 39-year-old man with diabetes. **(A)** CT demonstrates a filling defect within the left lower lobe pulmonary artery (*arrow*). **(B)** Lung windows demonstrate a large adjacent lung abscess.

A

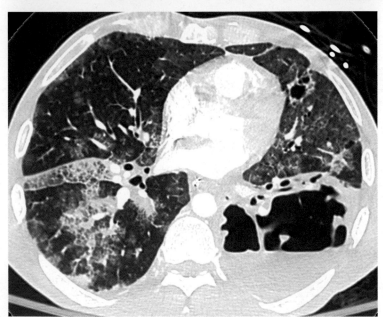

B

◆ Vasculitis-Related Pulmonary Artery Thrombosis

- ◆ Behçet syndrome, Hughes-Stovin syndrome, and Takayasu arteritis can cause a vasculitis of large to medium-sized arteries within the thorax.

- ◆ The associated vessel wall inflammation can manifest as vessel wall thickening and occlusive in situ thrombosis (**Fig. 5.6**).
- ◆ Although deep vein thrombosis is common, particularly in Behçet syndrome, pulmonary embolism is rare because the thrombi in the inflamed veins of the lower extremities are strongly adherent.

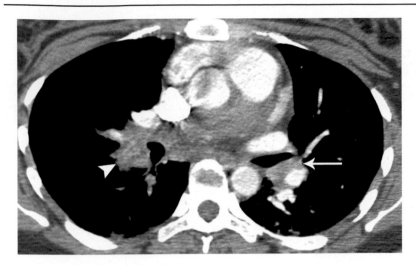

Fig. 5.6 Takayasu arteritis in a 28-year-old woman. Contrast material–enhanced CT demonstrates eccentric thickening of the left lower lobe pulmonary artery wall (*arrow*) and occlusion of the right lower lobe pulmonary artery (*arrowhead*).

◆ In Situ Thrombosis in Pulmonary Hypertension

- ◆ Pulmonary artery in situ thrombosis can be seen in any patient with pulmonary artery hypertension.
- ◆ A comprehensive list of causes is provided in Chapter 12 of this book.
- ◆ Congenital systemic-to-pulmonary shunts include ventricular septal defect, atrial septal defect, and patent ductus arteriosus, which can result in Eisenmenger syndrome.
- ◆ Eisenmenger syndrome is defined as the process in which a chronic left-to-right shunt in the heart results in pulmonary arterial hypertension. This in turn causes a reversal of blood flow and a right-to-left shunt.
- ◆ The prevalence of proximal pulmonary artery thrombus in Eisenmenger syndrome is approximately 25%. Such thrombi are often seen in aneurysms (**Fig. 5.7**).

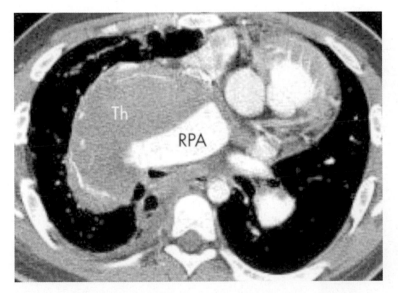

A

Fig. 5.7 (A,B) In situ pulmonary artery thrombosis in a 21-year-old man with atrioventricular septal defect and Eisenmenger syndrome. **(A)** Axial CT demonstrates a massively dilated right pulmonary artery (*RPA*) and a large in situ thrombus (*Th*). (Continued on page 88)

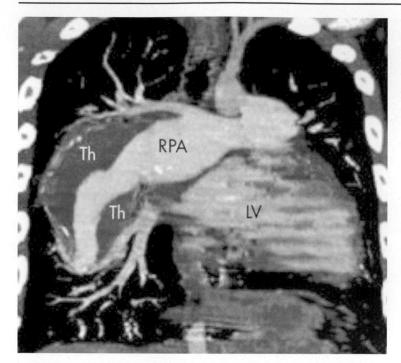

B

Fig. 5.7 (*Continued*) In situ pulmonary artery thrombosis in a 21-year-old man with atrioventricular septal defect and Eisenmenger syndrome. **(B)** Oblique coronal image shows the dilated right pulmonary artery (*RPA*) overlying the left ventricle (*LV*) and a large concentric thrombus (*Th*) adjacent to calcified atheroma. (Reproduced from Broberg C, Ujita M, Babu-Narayan S, et al. Massive pulmonary artery thrombosis with haemoptysis in adults with Eisenmenger's syndrome: a clinical dilemma. Heart 2004;90(11):e63, with permission from BMJ Publishing Group Ltd.)

◆ Pulmonary Vein Thrombosis

◆ In situ thrombosis of the pulmonary vein has been described in patients after thoracic surgery for lobectomy or lung transplant, radio-frequency ablation, or chest trauma. It has also been described in patients with left atrial dilatation and atrial fibrillation.

◆ This is a potentially devastating disease that can lead to peripheral arterial embolism with transient ischemic attacks and stroke.

◆ Diagnostic tools include computed tomography (CT; **Fig. 5.8**), magnetic resonance imaging, and transesophageal echocardiography.

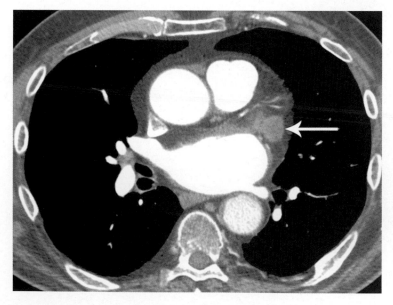

A

Fig. 5.8 (A,B) Pulmonary vein thrombosis in a 74-year-old woman with atrial fibrillation. **(A)** Thrombus is demonstrated in the left atrial appendage (*arrow*).

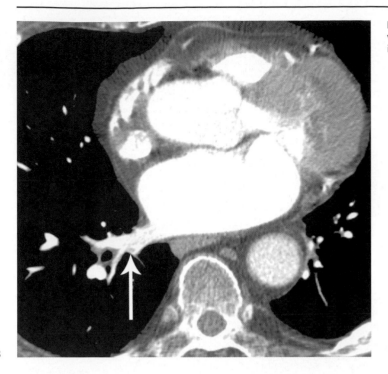

B

Fig. 5.8 (*Continued*) Pulmonary vein thrombosis in a 74-year-old woman with atrial fibrillation. **(B)** A small, well-defined thrombus is also seen in the right inferior pulmonary vein (*arrow*).

◆ Pulmonary Vein Thrombosis Mimic on Computed Tomography

◆ In general, CT acquires one time point of the pulmonary veins.

◆ Opacification of the pulmonary vein depends on the timing of the contrast material injection.

◆ The pulmonary artery–to–pulmonary vein transit time can be delayed by a large pulmonary artery thomboembolism or by an increase in vascular resistance due to atelectasis or consolidation.

◆ Unopacified blood can mimic thrombus. Such a flow artifact classically has ill-defined margins (**Fig. 5.9**).

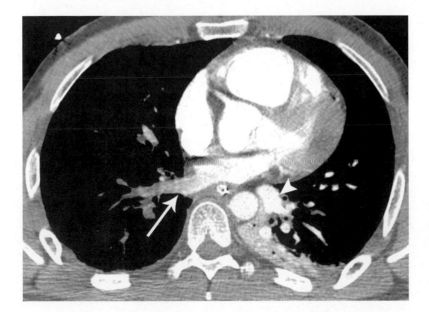

Fig. 5.9 Poor vein opacification in a 30-year-old man with massive right acute thromboembolism. On CT, extensive emboli are seen in the middle and right lower lobe pulmonary arteries. As a consequence of the different flow rates of contrast material, at this stage there is good enhancement of the left inferior pulmonary vein (*arrowhead*) and poor enhancement of the right inferior pulmonary vein, demonstrated by an ill-defined interface between poorly opacified and well-opacified blood (*arrow*).

Suggested Reading

Brown JM, Farjardo LF, Stewart JR. Mural thrombosis of the heart induced by radiation. Arch Pathol 1973;96(1):1–4

Burri E, Duwe J, Kull C, Glaser C, Maurer CA. Pulmonary vein thrombosis after lower lobectomy of the left lung. J Cardiovasc Surg (Torino) 2006;47(5):609–612

Doust BC, Rathe JW. Main branch pulmonary artery thrombosis with pulmonary abscess formation: case report. Ann Intern Med 1958; 48(1):170–174

Garcia MJ, Rodriguez L, Vandervoort P. Pulmonary vein thrombosis and peripheral embolization. Chest 1996;109(3):846–847

Girod JP, Lopez-Candales A. Pulmonary vein thrombosis in the setting of blunt chest trauma. J Am Soc Echocardiogr 2007;20(12):1416, e1

Girinsky T. [Effects of ionizing radiation on the blood vessel wall]. J Mal Vasc 2000;25(5):321–324

Hiller N, Lieberman S, Chajek-Shaul T, Bar-Ziv J, Shaham D. Thoracic manifestations of Behçet disease at CT. Radiographics 2004;24(3):801–808

Kwek BH, Wittram C. Postpneumonectomy pulmonary artery stump thrombosis: CT features and imaging follow-up. Radiology 2005; 237(1):338–341

Luna CM, Baquero S, Gando S, et al. Experimental severe pseudomonas aeruginosa pneumonia and antibiotic therapy in piglets receiving mechanical ventilation. Chest 2007;132(2):523–531

Perloff JK, Rosove MH, Child JS, Wright GB. Adults with cyanotic congenital heart disease: hematologic management. Ann Intern Med 1988; 109(5):406–413

Schulman LL, Anandarangam T, Leibowitz DW, et al. Four-year prospective study of pulmonary venous thrombosis after lung transplantation. J Am Soc Echocardiogr 2001;14(8):806–812

Silversides CK, Granton JT, Konen E, Hart MA, Webb GD, Therrien J. Pulmonary thrombosis in adults with Eisenmenger syndrome. J Am Coll Cardiol 2003;42(11):1982–1987

Uzun O, Akpolat T, Erkan L. Pulmonary vasculitis in Behçet disease: a cumulative analysis. Chest 2005;127(6):2243–2253

Virchow R. Cellular pathology as based upon physiological and pathological histology. London, England: Churchill; 1860.

Wittram C, Maher MM, Yoo AJ, Kalra MK, Shepard JA, McLoud TC. CT angiography of pulmonary embolism: diagnostic criteria and causes of misdiagnosis. Radiographics 2004;24(5):1219–1238

Wnuk-Wojnar AM, Trusz-Gluza M, Czerwiński C, et al. Circumferential pulmonary vein RF ablation in the treatment of atrial fibrillation: 3-year experience of one centre. Kardiol Pol 2005;63(4):362–370, discussion 371–372

6

Aneurysm and Varix

An aneurysm is a focal widening of an artery. A true aneurysm contains all three major layers: adventitia, media, and intima. In a false aneurysm, or pseudoaneurysm, one or more of these layers is missing. True aneurysms can be fusiform or saccular in shape; false aneurysms tend to be saccular. A pulmonary artery aneurysm can be congenital or acquired. Although pulmonary artery aneurysms are infrequent, the main causes include trauma, catheter injury, infections, vasculitis, pulmonary hypertension, neoplasms, and connective tissue disorders (Marfan syndrome); pulmonary artery aneurysms may also be idiopathic. Aneurysms can progress to pulmonary artery dissection or rupture, particularly large aneurysms with associated pulmonary artery hypertension. Post-stenotic dilatation of a pulmonary artery can be seen distal to pulmonary valve stenosis. Bronchial artery aneurysm is uncommon; the etiologic factors are the same as for any systemic artery aneurysm, and similarly, rupture can have a devastating effect. Pulmonary vein varices may be congenital or associated with chronic pulmonary venous hypertension; these dilated veins tend to have a benign course. In this chapter, examples of pulmonary and bronchial artery aneurysms and pulmonary vein varix are illustrated.

◆ Fusiform Aneurysms

- *Fusiform aneurysm* is a descriptive term for a focal, concentric, symmetric widening of an artery (**Fig. 6.1**).

◆ Saccular Aneurysms

- *Saccular aneurysm* is a descriptive term for a focal, eccentrically located, asymmetric widening of an artery (**Fig. 6.2**).
- Mycotic, traumatic, and catheter injury–induced aneurysms tend to be saccular in shape.

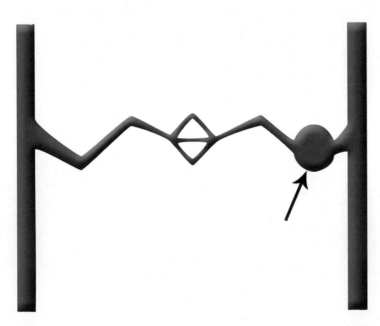

Fig. 6.1 Illustration of fusiform aneurysm. There is a focal, concentric, symmetric widening of the vessel (*arrow*).

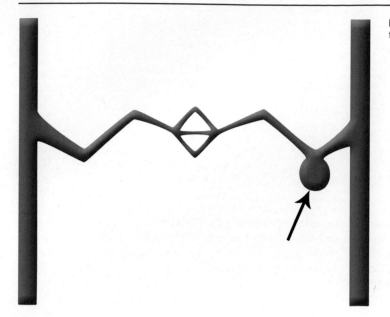

Fig. 6.2 Illustration of saccular aneurysm. There is a focal, eccentric, asymmetric widening of the vessel (*arrow*).

◆ **Post-Stenotic Dilatation of the Pulmonary Artery**

- ◆ This can occur distal to pulmonary valve stenosis.
- ◆ The dilatation is usually congenital but can occur in carcinoid syndrome or as a result of rheumatic fever.
- ◆ There is obstruction to right ventricular outflow.
- ◆ The jet through the stenosed valve dilates the main and/or left pulmonary artery (**Fig. 6.3**).
- ◆ The right pulmonary artery classically remains normal in size.

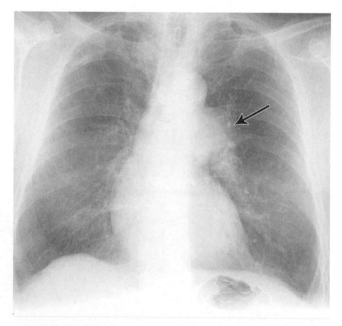

A

Fig. 6.3 (A–C) Pulmonary valve stenosis in a 75-year-old man. **(A)** Chest radiograph demonstrates left pulmonary artery enlargement (*arrow*).

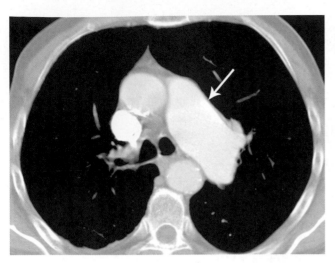

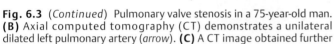

B

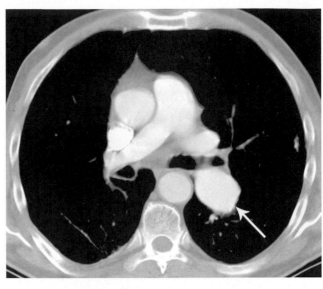

C

Fig. 6.3 (*Continued*) Pulmonary valve stenosis in a 75-year-old man. **(B)** Axial computed tomography (CT) demonstrates a unilateral dilated left pulmonary artery (*arrow*). **(C)** A CT image obtained further caudad shows the normally sized main and right pulmonary arteries and the dilated left pulmonary artery (*arrow*).

◆ **Pulmonary Artery Injury**

◆ One iatrogenic cause is a poorly positioned pulmonary artery catheter, with the tip placed too peripherally.
◆ The catheter tip can erode the artery wall and result in a pseudoaneurysm, which is often saccular (**Fig. 6.4**).
◆ The incidence of pulmonary artery rupture resulting from pulmonary artery catheter insertion is 0.03%, with a 70% mortality rate.
◆ Other causes of pulmonary artery injury include chest tube insertion, angiography, surgical resection, lung biopsy, and penetrating trauma from stab or gunshot wounds.

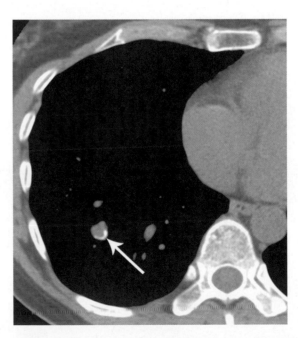

A

Fig. 6.4 (A–C) Pulmonary artery saccular aneurysm in a 48-year-old man after remote pulmonary artery catheterization. **(A)** Non–contrast-enhanced CT demonstrates a nodular opacity in the right lower lobe with some curvilinear wall calcification (*arrow*). (*Continued on page 94*)

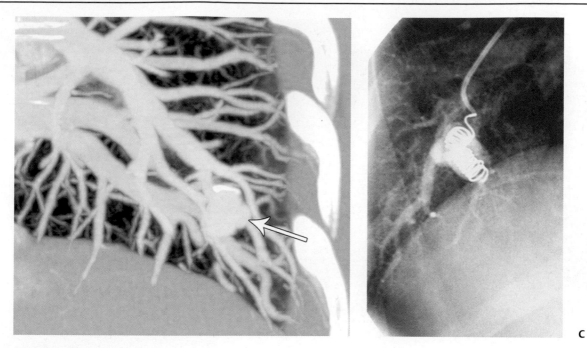

Fig. 6.4 (*Continued*) Pulmonary artery saccular aneurysm in a 48-year-old man after remote pulmonary artery catheterization. **(B)** Contrast material–enhanced CT maximum-intensity projection (MIP) image demonstrates the pseudoaneurysm arising from a subsegmental artery of the right lower lobe (*arrow*). **(C)** Spot image of an angiogram demonstrates coil placement into the saccular aneurysm.

◆ Mycotic Aneurysm

- ◆ Mycotic aneurysm can result from bacterial (**Fig. 6.5**), fungal, or mycobacterial infection. (An aneurysm due to tuberculosis is known as a Rasmussen aneurysm).
- ◆ Mycotic aneurysms tend to be pseudoaneurysms and carry a risk for pulmonary hemorrhage and life-threatening hemoptysis.

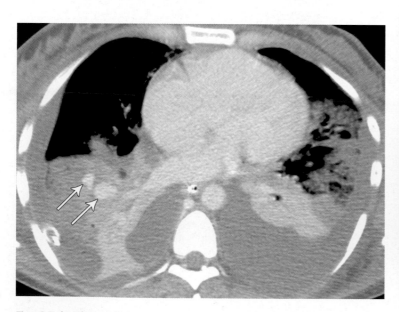
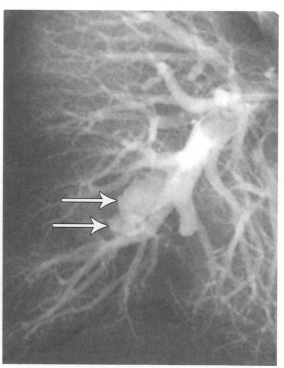

Fig. 6.5 (A,B) Pseudoaneurysms in a 36-year-old female drug addict with staphylococcal pneumonia. **(A)** CT demonstrates two saccular aneurysms in the right lower lobe (*arrows*). **(B)** Angiogram confirms the two pseudoaneurysms (*arrows*). Occluded arteries are also seen.

◆ Tumor Aneurysm

- ◆ Primary lung cancer (**Fig. 6.6**), pulmonary metastases, and less commonly tumors arising from the pulmonary arteries can erode the pulmonary arteries and result in a pseudoaneurysm.
- ◆ There is a large risk for life-threatening massive hemoptysis.

◆ Vasculitic Aneurysm

- ◆ Behçet syndrome and Hughes-Stovin syndrome are the most common vasculitic diseases associated with pulmonary artery aneurysms (**Fig. 6.7**).
- ◆ Behçet syndrome is a chronic multisystem vasculitis characterized by recurrent oral and genital ulcers and uveitis.
- ◆ The pulmonary artery aneurysms in Behçet syndrome may regress with immunosuppressive therapy. However, embolization may be necessary.
- ◆ Behçet syndrome includes vascular thrombosis, pulmonary infarction, and hemorrhage.
- ◆ Hughes-Stovin syndrome may present with recurrent thrombophlebitis and pulmonary artery aneurysm formation and rupture. It is considered by some to be a forme fruste of Behçet syndrome.

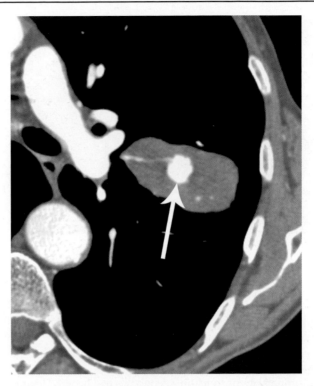

Fig. 6.6 Pseudoaneurysm in a 61-year-old man with poorly differentiated non–small-cell lung cancer. CT demonstrates a pulmonary artery aneurysm arising within the middle of the necrotic lung neoplasm (*arrow*).

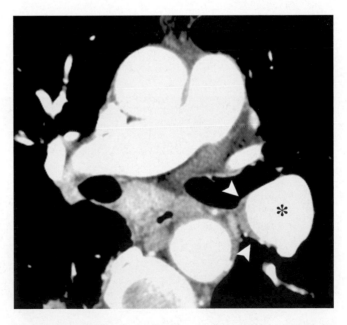

Fig. 6.7 Behçet disease in a 50-year-old man with hemoptysis. CT scan shows aneurysmal dilatation of a left interlobar pulmonary artery (*) with medial mural thickening (*arrowheads*). (Reproduced with permission from author and publisher: Castañer E, Gallardo X, Rimola J, et al. Congenital and acquired pulmonary artery anomalies in the adult: radiologic overview. Radiographics 2006;26:349–371.)

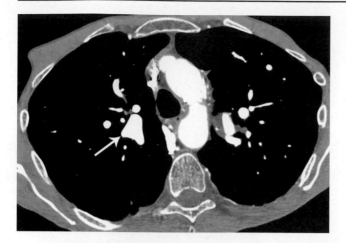

Fig. 6.8 Chronic thrombotic pulmonary embolism and pulmonary artery hypertension in a 60-year-old man. CT at the level of the upper lobes demonstrates a fusiform pulmonary artery aneurysm at a branch point on the right (*arrow*).

◆ Pulmonary Hypertension

- ◆ Pulmonary arterial hypertension is a common cause of pulmonary artery aneurysm.
- ◆ A comprehensive list of causes is provided in Chapter 12 of this book.
- ◆ Pulmonary hypertension secondary to chronic thrombotic embolic disease is one of the more common causes (**Fig. 6.8**).

◆ Idiopathic Aneurysm

- ◆ By definition, a pulmonary artery aneurysm is idiopathic when all known causes have been excluded.
- ◆ Large aneurysms can become symptomatic due to the local compression of adjacent structures.
- ◆ Pulmonary valve insufficiency and right ventricular dysfunction can occur.
- ◆ Because of the risk for rupture, idiopathic aneurysms are often treated surgically when larger than 6 cm (**Fig. 6.9**).

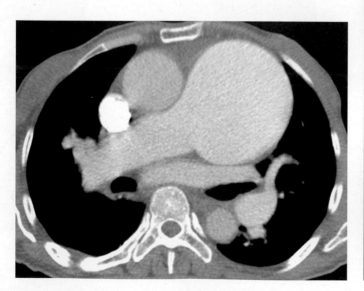

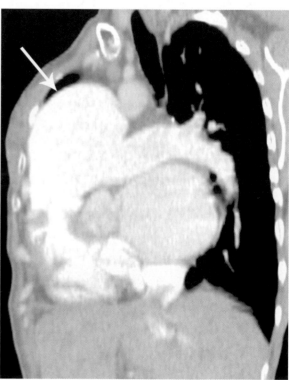

A

B

Fig. 6.9 (A,B) Idiopathic pulmonary artery aneurysms in a 63-year-old woman. (A) CT demonstrates hugely dilated main and left pulmonary arteries. (B) Sagittal oblique image shows the aneurysm as a saccular bulge arising from the main and left pulmonary arteries superiorly (*arrow*).

◆ Bronchial Artery Aneurysm

- ◆ Bronchial artery aneurysms most often occur in patients with predisposing pulmonary disease, including bronchiectasis, lung cancer, and recurrent infection.
- ◆ They are classified anatomically as either mediastinal (**Fig. 6.10**) or intrapulmonary.
- ◆ A mediastinal aneurysm may mimic an aortic aneurysm or dissection and can manifest as a mediastinal mass, superior vena cava obstruction, dysphagia, hemothorax, hemomediastinum, or hematemesis.
- ◆ Intrapulmonary aneurysms may present with massive or intermittent hemoptysis.
- ◆ Early diagnosis and treatment are crucial because of the possibility of life-threatening rupture and hemorrhage.

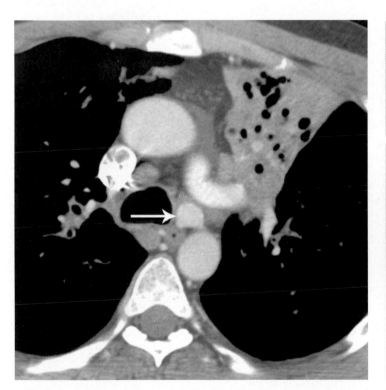

A

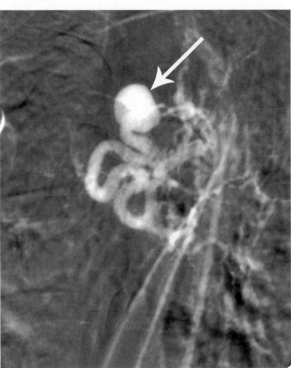

B

Fig. 6.10 (A,B) Bronchial artery aneurysm in a 36-year-old man with cystic fibrosis. **(A)** CT demonstrates a saccular aneurysm arising from the bronchial artery near its origin from the descending aorta (*arrow*). **(B)** Bronchial artery angiogram before coiling demonstrates the aneurysm (*arrow*).

◆ Pulmonary Vein Varix

- ◆ A pulmonary vein varix can be congenital or acquired as a consequence of chronic pulmonary venous hypertension.
- ◆ It most often presents as an asymptomatic, well-defined mediastinal or lung mass on chest radiography.
- ◆ Treatment is usually unnecessary once the vascular nature of the lesion has been recognized (**Fig. 6.11**).
- ◆ Exceedingly rare complications include systemic embolization secondary to thrombus in the varix and rupture of the varix into the pleural space or into a bronchus with hemoptysis.

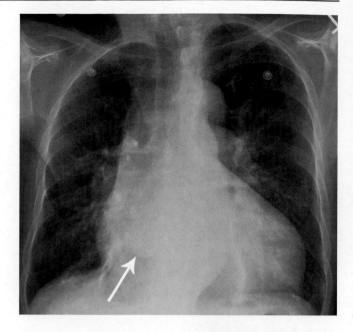

A

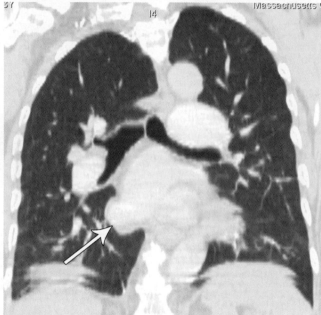

B

Fig. 6.11 (A,B) Pulmonary vein varix in a 76-year-old man. **(A)** Frontal chest radiograph shows a smooth, nodular opacity behind the right side of the heart (*arrow*). **(B)** CT coronal reconstruction MIP image demonstrates a pulmonary varix affecting the right inferior pulmonary vein (*arrow*).

Suggested Reading

Deb SJ, Zehr KJ, Shields RC. Idiopathic pulmonary artery aneurysm. Ann Thorac Surg 2005;80(4):1500–1502

Gomez-Jorge J, Mitchell SE. Embolization of a pulmonary artery pseudoaneurysm due to squamous cell carcinoma of the lung. J Vasc Interv Radiol 1999;10(8):1127–1130

Graham JK, Shehata B. Sudden death due to dissecting pulmonary artery aneurysm: a case report and review of the literature. Am J Forensic Med Pathol 2007;28(4):342–344

Nair KKS, Cobanoglu AM. Idiopathic main pulmonary artery aneurysm. Ann Thorac Surg 2001;71(5):1688–1690

Nguyen ET, Silva CIS, Seely JM, Chong S, Lee KS, Müller NL. Pulmonary artery aneurysms and pseudoaneurysms in adults: findings at CT and radiography. AJR Am J Roentgenol 2007;188(2):W126–134

Vanherreweghe E, Rigauts H, Bogaerts Y, Meeus L. Pulmonary vein varix: diagnosis with multi-slice helical CT. Eur Radiol 2000;10(8):1315–1317

Wilson SR, Winger DI, Katz DS. CT visualization of mediastinal bronchial artery aneurysm. AJR Am J Roentgenol 2006;187(5):W544–W545

Yoon W, Kim JK, Kim YH, Chung TW, Kang HK. Bronchial and nonbronchial systemic artery embolization for life-threatening hemoptysis: a comprehensive review. Radiographics 2002;22(6):1395–1409

7

Vasculitis

The vasculitides are a diverse group of diseases characterized by inflammation within and around blood vessel walls. This inflammatory process can affect large and medium-size vessels as well as small vessels and capillaries that are below the resolution of computed tomography (CT). Behçet syndrome, Hughes-Stovin syndrome, Takayasu arteritis, and giant cell arteritis tend to affect the large and medium-size arteries, whereas Wegener granulomatosis, microscopic polyangiitis, Churg-Strauss syndrome, Goodpasture syndrome, cryoglobulinemia, Henoch-Schönlein purpura, connective tissue diseases, and drug-induced vasculitis tend to involve small pulmonary vessels and capillaries. The vasculitides can also be classified according to histologic patterns. For example, giant cell infiltrate is seen in giant cell arteritis and Takayasu arteritis; granulomatous infiltrate in Wegener granulomatosis, microscopic polyangiitis, and Churg-Strauss syndrome; leukocytoclastic infiltrate in cryoglobulinemia, Henoch-Schönlein purpura, and Behçet syndrome; and lymphocytic infiltrate in connective tissue, Behçet syndrome, and drug-induced vasculitides. Goodpasture syndrome, Wegener granulomatosis, microscopic polyangiitis, Churg-Strauss syndrome, and systemic lupus erythematosus are all possible causes of the pulmonary-renal syndrome. The most common respiratory symptom of the pulmonary vasculitides is hemoptysis, which can be life-threatening. This chapter summarizes the pulmonary vasculitides and illustrates the imaging findings.

◆ Behçet Syndrome

- Behçet syndrome is a chronic multisystem vasculitis characterized by recurrent oral and genital ulcers and uveitis.
- It occurs most commonly in Turkey and Southeast Asia and is associated with human leukocyte antigen B51 and with *Staphylococcus aureus*, *Prevotella*, *Chlamydia*, and hepatitis C infections.
- Thoracic manifestations include arterial aneurysms (**Fig. 7.1**), vascular thrombosis, pulmonary infarction, hemorrhage, organizing pneumonia, lymphadenopathy, and pleural effusion.
- The pulmonary artery aneurysms in Behçet syndrome may regress with immunosuppressive therapy. However, embolization may be necessary.

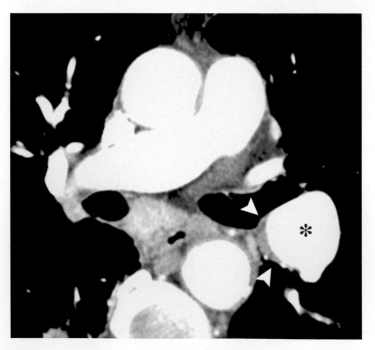

Fig. 7.1 Behçet syndrome in a 50-year-old man with hemoptysis. CT scan shows aneurysmal dilatation of a left interlobar pulmonary artery (*) with medial mural thickening (*arrowheads*). (Reproduced with permission from author and publisher: Castañer E, Gallardo X, Rimola J, et al. Congenital and acquired pulmonary artery anomalies in the adult: radiologic overview. Radiographics 2006;26(2): 349–371.)

- It is important that pulmonary vasculitis is not mistaken for pulmonary thromboembolic disease because fatalities have occurred shortly after the initiation of anticoagulation.
- Hughes-Stovin syndrome may present with recurrent thrombophlebitis and pulmonary artery aneurysm formation and rupture. It is considered by some to be a forme fruste of Behçet syndrome.

- Pulmonary vascular changes include wall thickening, in situ thrombosis, stenosis, occlusion (**Fig. 7.2**), and pulmonary hypertension.
- Organization of thrombosis and recanalization occur; the new vessels are often vasa vasorum that are branches of the bronchial artery.
- Mosaic attenuation and peripheral lung nodules (**Fig. 7.2C**) have been described, indicative of involvement of small pulmonary arteries and adjacent lung tissue.

◆ Takayasu Arteritis

- Takayasu arteritis is a chronic, progressive systemic arteritis of unknown cause that classically involves the aorta and its branches.
- It is most common in East Asia, affecting women of childbearing age.
- Pulmonary vascular involvement occurs in 50 to 80% of cases.

◆ Giant Cell Arteritis

- Giant cell arteritis is an idiopathic vasculitis that involves large arteries, predominantly the extracranial carotid branches and the aorta; it rarely involves central pulmonary arteries.
- The classic clinical picture is a woman older than 50 years with polymyalgia rheumatica, headache, systemic illness, and a high erythrocyte sedimentation rate.

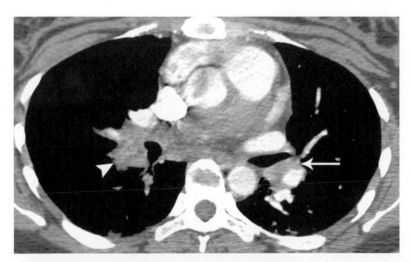

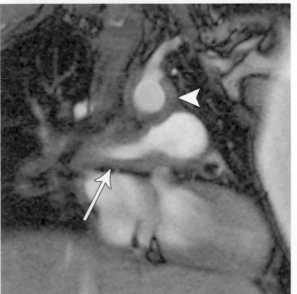

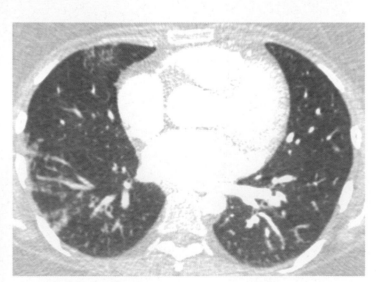

Fig. 7.2 (A–C) Takayasu arteritis in a 28-year-old woman. **(A)** CT demonstrates eccentric enhancing wall thickening of the left lower lobe pulmonary artery (*arrow*) and occlusion of the right lower lobe pulmonary artery (*arrowhead*). **(B)** Contrast material–enhanced magnetic resonance image (MRI) demonstrates wall thickening and enhancement of the right lower lobe pulmonary artery (*arrow*) just before the obstruction. There is also involvement of the aorta (*arrowhead*). **(C)** CT on lung windows shows subpleural and peribronchovascular nodules affecting the right lung.

A

B

C

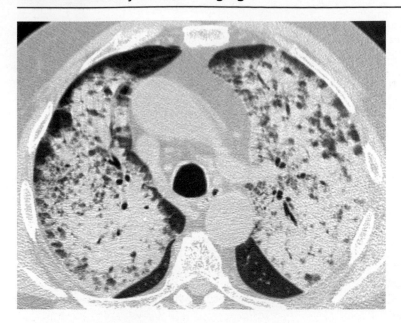

Fig. 7.3 Wegener granulomatosis in an 83-year-old man. High-resolution CT of the upper lobes demonstrates diffuse bilateral consolidation, consistent with diffuse pulmonary hemorrhage.

- The CT features of giant cell arteritis of the pulmonary arteries are similar to those of Takayasu arteritis, with arterial wall thickening, stenosis, and in situ thrombosis.

◆ Wegener Granulomatosis

- Wegener granulomatosis is an idiopathic inflammatory systemic disease characterized by a necrotizing granulomatous vasculitis of the upper and lower respiratory tract, focal necrotizing glomerulonephritis, and vasculitis affecting small arteries, capillaries, and veins.

- It may also affect the joints, eyes, nervous system, heart, gastrointestinal tract, thyroid gland, liver, and breasts.
- The mean age at onset is the fifth decade.
- Notable laboratory findings are positivity for c-ANCA (circulating anti-neutrophil cytoplasmic antibody) and anti-PR3 (anti-proteinase 3) in 90% of cases, with a high erythrocyte sedimentation rate.
- Several patterns of Wegener granulomatosis can affect the thorax: diffuse alveolar hemorrhage (**Fig. 7.3**), the typical cavitary nodules or masses (**Figs. 7.4** and **7.5**), and less commonly large vessel disease (**Fig. 7.6**).

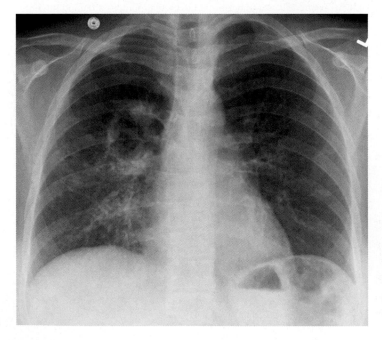

A

Fig. 7.4 (A,B) Wegener granulomatosis in a 23-year-old woman. **(A)** Frontal chest radiograph demonstrates a large cavitary mass in the right lung adjacent to the hilum. In addition, there are ill-defined small nodular opacities in the middle and lower lung regions bilaterally, consistent with aspirated blood.

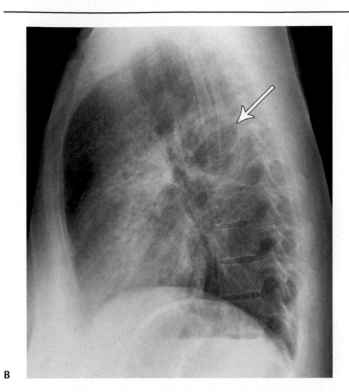

B

Fig. 7.4 (*Continued*) Wegener granulomatosis in a 23-year-old woman. **(B)** Lateral radiograph demonstrates that the large cavitary mass is located in the superior segment of the right lower lobe (*arrow*). Consolidation anterior to the cavitary mass is likely related to pulmonary hemorrhage.

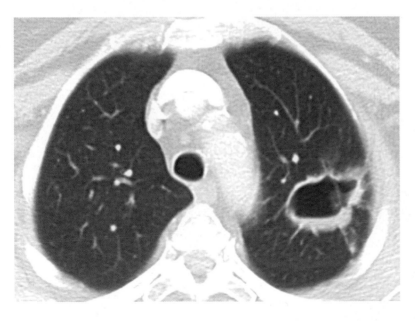

Fig. 7.5 Wegener granulomatosis in a 68-year-old woman. CT shows the classic cavitary mass of Wegener granulomatosis in the left upper lobe.

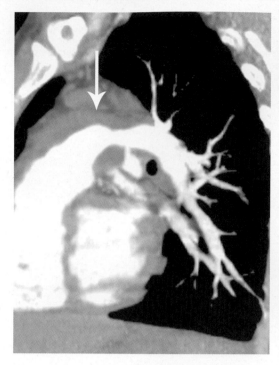

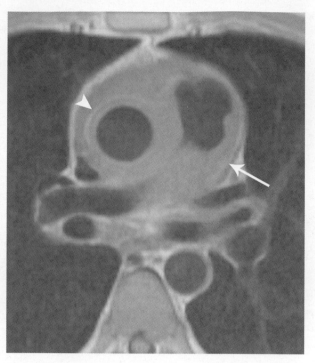

A   B

Fig. 7.6 (A,B) Wegener granulomatosis in a 39-year-old man. **(A)** Oblique sagittal contrast-enhanced CT demonstrates concentric asymmetric wall thickening of the left pulmonary artery (*arrow*). **(B)** Axial contrast-enhanced MRI demonstrates concentric wall thickening and enhancement of the aorta (*arrowhead*) and concentric nodular asymmetric wall thickening of the left pulmonary artery (*arrow*). Incidental note is made of left main bronchus wall thickening.

◆ Microscopic Polyangiitis

◆ Microscopic polyangiitis is a nongranulomatous necrotizing systemic vasculitis that affects arterioles, capillaries, venules, and on occasion medium-size vessels. Glomerulonephritis is almost always present.

◆ It tends to affect men 55 to 74 years of age; an association with exposure to silica, solvents, and medicines has been suggested.

◆ Patients are often positive for p-ANCA (perinuclear antineutrophil cytoplasmic antibody); they may also be positive for c-ANCA.

◆ Recurring diffuse alveolar hemorrhage is common, seen in 30 to 40% of patients.

◆ The imaging appearance at presentation is that of diffuse alveolar hemorrhage (**Fig. 7.7**). In the stationary clinical phases, CT may show centrilobular ground-glass nodules, representing perivascular inflammation (**Fig. 7.8**), or diffuse interstitial fibrosis.

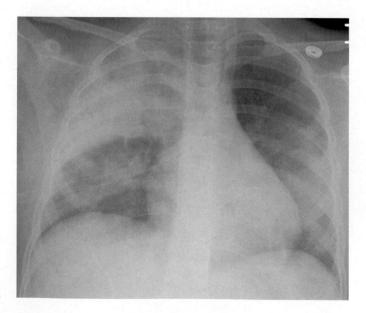

A

Fig. 7.7 (A,B) Microscopic polyangiitis in a 7-year-old girl. **(A)** Admission chest radiograph demonstrates extensive bilateral consolidation with some sparing of the left upper lobe.

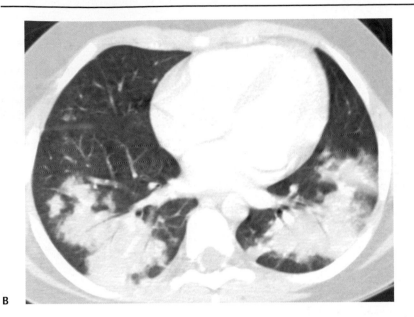

B

Fig. 7.7 (*Continued*) Microscopic polyangiitis in a 7-year-old girl. **(B)** CT demonstrates bilateral lower lobe consolidation, consistent with pulmonary hemorrhage.

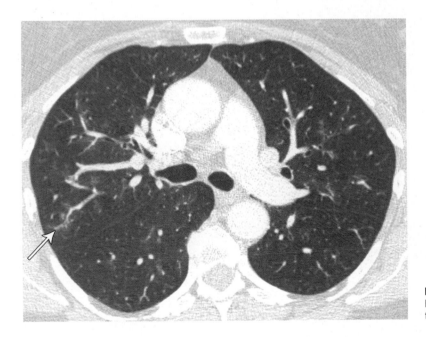

Fig. 7.8 Microscopic polyangiitis in a 55-year-old woman. High-resolution CT demonstrates ground-glass opacities that have a peribronchovascular distribution (*arrow*).

◆ Churg-Strauss Syndrome

- ◆ Churg-Strauss syndrome is a systemic disease associated with p-ANCA.
- ◆ Clinically, three phases occur: a prodromal phase of asthma and allergic rhinitis, an eosinophilic phase of peripheral blood eosinophilia and eosinophilic tissue infiltrates, and a vasculitic phase of life-threatening systemic vasculitis of small and medium-size vessels associated with vascular and extravascular granulomatosis.
- ◆ Other manifestations include segmental glomerulonephritis, peripheral neuropathy, cardiomyopathy, purpuric rash, and abdominal pain.

- ◆ The eosinophilic phase is characterized by transient migratory pulmonary consolidation on chest radiography due to eosinophilic pneumonia (**Fig. 7.9A**).
- ◆ The vasculitic phase may present with consolidation or ground-glass opacification due to pulmonary hemorrhage.
- ◆ CT findings vary according to the stage of disease and include the following: consolidation and ground-glass opacities, which may be peripheral (**Fig. 7.9B**); pulmonary centrilobular nodules; interlobular septal thickening; bronchial wall thickening; and bronchiectasis.

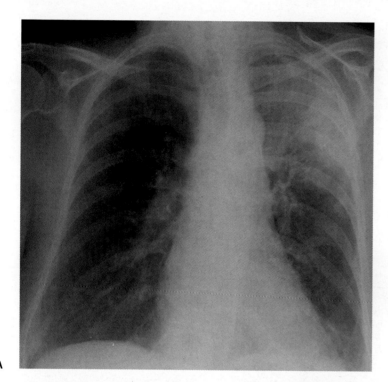

A

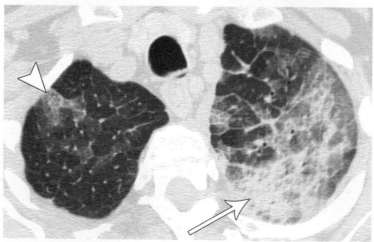

B

Fig. 7.9 (A,B) Churg-Strauss syndrome in a 69-year-old woman. **(A)** Chest radiograph demonstrates peripheral consolidation in the left upper lobe and subtle ground-glass opacification of the lower lobes. **(B)** High-resolution CT demonstrates peripheral consolidation (*arrow*) and peripheral ground-glass opacification with diffuse interlobular septal thickening and intralobular interstitial thickening (*arrowhead*).

◆ Goodpasture Syndrome

- ◆ Goodpasture syndrome is an antiglomerular basement membrane antibody disease.
- ◆ A patchy linear deposition of immunoglobulin is found along the alveolar basement membranes.
- ◆ Lung biopsy specimens usually show intra-alveolar hemorrhage and hemosiderin deposition.

- ◆ The disease presents most often in young adult men in association with dry cough, hemoptysis, and laboratory evidence of renal disease.
- ◆ The radiographic appearance is that of diffuse air space consolidation (**Fig. 7.10**).

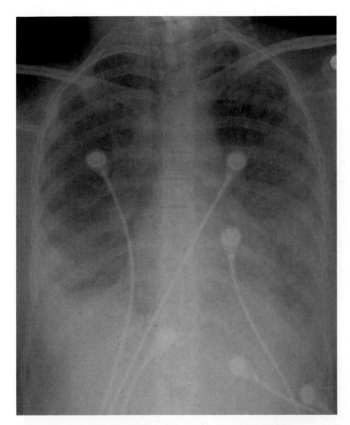

A

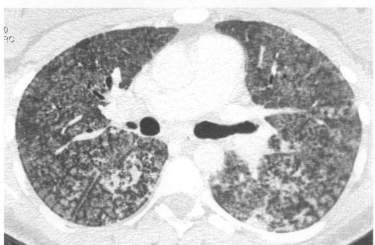

B

Fig. 7.10 (A,B) Goodpasture syndrome in a 26-year-old woman. **(A)** Chest radiograph on admission demonstrates bilateral diffuse ground-glass opacification and bilateral lower lobe consolidation. **(B)** High-resolution CT shows predominantly centrilobular ground-glass opacities, some forming a rosette pattern.

◆ Cryoglobulinemic Vasculitis

- ◆ Cryoglobulins are immunoglobulins that precipitate on exposure to cold.
- ◆ Vasculitis is caused by the deposition of mixed cryoglobulins in vessel walls, which results in acute inflammation.
- ◆ The average age of patients is approximately 50 years.
- ◆ An associated hepatitis C virus infection is seen in 80% of cases and is thought to be an etiologic factor.
- ◆ Clinical features include purpura, arthralgia, distal necroses, peripheral neuropathy, abdominal pain, and glomerulonephritis.
- ◆ It rarely manifests as diffuse pulmonary hemorrhage.

◆ Henoch-Schönlein Purpura

- ◆ Henoch-Schönlein purpura is the most common systemic vasculitis in children; the peak incidence is at 5 years of age.
- ◆ It is characterized by the deposition of mainly immunoglobulin A and immunoglobulin C3 immune complexes in various organs.
- ◆ It can present with characteristic nonthrombocytopenic purpura, arthralgia, abdominal pain associated with intussusception, glomerulonephritis, and occasionally pulmonary hemorrhage (**Fig. 7.11**).
- ◆ Diffuse pulmonary hemorrhage, when it occurs, is more common in adults than in children.

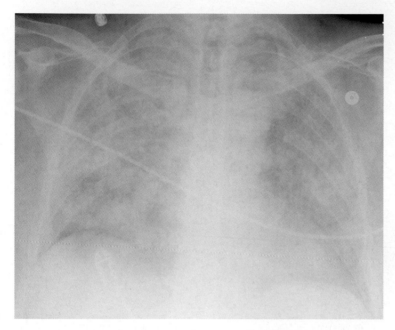

A

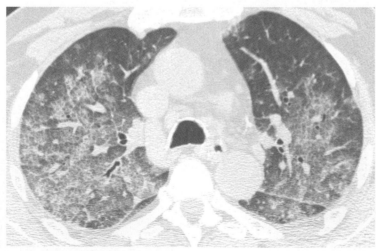

B

Fig. 7.11 (A,B) Henoch-Schönlein purpura in a 23-year-old man. **(A)** Admission chest radiograph demonstrates diffuse bilateral ground-glass opacification and consolidation. **(B)** High-resolution CT demonstrates diffuse bilateral ground-glass opacification, interlobular septal thickening, and intralobular interstitial thickening ("crazy paving"), consistent with diffuse pulmonary hemorrhage.

◆ Systemic Lupus Erythematosus

◆ Diffuse pulmonary hemorrhage can occur in any collagen-vascular disease, but it is most commonly seen in systemic lupus erythematosus (SLE).

◆ Most patients with pulmonary hemorrhage in association with SLE have an established diagnosis of multisystem SLE; in rare cases, pulmonary hemorrhage may be the first manifestation of SLE (**Fig. 7.12**).

◆ Neutrophilic alveolar capillaritis is the most common histologic lesion causing pulmonary hemorrhage in patients with SLE.

◆ The diagnosis of SLE is established by the detection of serum antinuclear antibodies.

◆ High-resolution CT lung changes of SLE include intralobular interstitial thickening, irregular interlobular septal thickening, and bronchiectasis and bronchiolectasis in a peripheral distribution.

◆ Drug-Induced Vasculitis

◆ Diffuse pulmonary hemorrhage can occur as a result of anticoagulant and thrombolytic therapy, the direct toxic effects of chemotherapeutic agents and "crack" cocaine, or a hypersensitivity reaction.

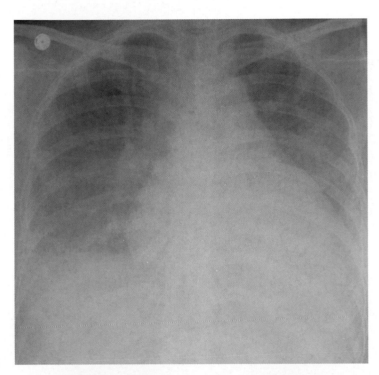

A

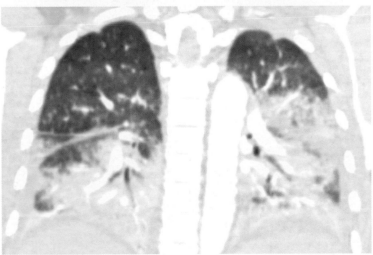

B

Fig. 7.12 (A–C) Systemic lupus erythematosus in a 23-year-old woman who presented with hemoptysis. **(A)** Portable chest radiograph demonstrates bilateral ground-glass and consolidation opacities in the middle and lower lung regions. **(B)** Coronal reconstruction CT shows bilateral lower lung and left midlung consolidation and upper lobe ground-glass opacification, consistent with pulmonary hemorrhage. (Continued on page 110)

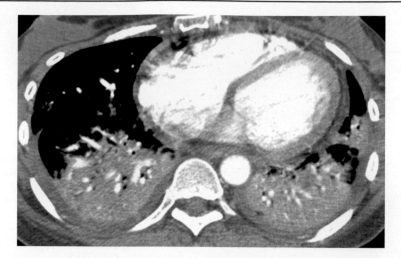

C

Fig. 7.12 (*Continued*) Systemic lupus erythematosus in a 23-year-old woman who presented with hemoptysis. **(C)** Axial CT of lung bases demonstrates bilateral lower lobe and lingular consolidation with small pleural and pericardial effusions.

◆ Drugs known to cause vasculitis include propyl-thiouracil, d-penicillamine, hydralazine, sulfasalazine, minocycline, allopurinol, all-*trans*-retinoic acid, penicillins, and leukotriene antagonists.

Suggested Reading

Clark T, Hoffman GS. Pulmonary artery involvement in Wegener's granulomatosis. Clin Exp Rheumatol 2003;21(6 Suppl 32):S124–S126

Fenlon HM, Doran M, Sant SM, Breatnach E. High-resolution chest CT in systemic lupus erythematosus. AJR Am J Roentgenol 1996;166(2): 301–307

Frankel SK, Cosgrove GP, Fischer A, Meehan RT, Brown KK. Update in the diagnosis and management of pulmonary vasculitis. Chest 2006; 129(2):452–465

Hansell DM. Small-vessel diseases of the lung: CT-pathologic correlates. Radiology 2002;225(3):639–653

Jennette JC, Falk RJ. Small-vessel vasculitis. N Engl J Med 1997;337(21): 1512–1523

Marten K, Schnyder P, Schirg E, Prokop M, Rummeny EJ, Engelke C. Pattern-based differential diagnosis in pulmonary vasculitis using volumetric CT. AJR Am J Roentgenol 2005;184(3):720–733

Nadrous HF, Yu AC, Specks U, Ryu JH. Pulmonary involvement in Henoch-Schönlein purpura. Mayo Clin Proc 2004;79(9):1151–1157

Paul JF, Hernigou A, Lefebvre C, et al. Electron beam CT features of the pulmonary artery in Takayasu's arteritis. AJR Am J Roentgenol 1999; 173(1):89–93

Primack SL, Miller RR, Müller NL. Diffuse pulmonary hemorrhage: clinical, pathologic, and imaging features. AJR Am J Roentgenol 1995;164(2): 295–300

Uzun O, Akpolat T, Erkan L. Pulmonary vasculitis in Behçet disease: a cumulative analysis. Chest 2005;127(6):2243–2253

Worthy SA, Müller NL, Hansell DM, Flower CD. Churg-Strauss syndrome: the spectrum of pulmonary CT findings in 17 patients. AJR Am J Roentgenol 1998;170(2):297–300

Yang CD, Teng JL, Gu YY, Chen SL. Takayasu's arteritis presenting with bilateral pulmonary granulomatosis. Clin Rheumatol 2007;26(4):612–614

8

Infection

Within this chapter, the manifestations of how pulmonary vessels can be a vector in the spread of infection to the lungs or be secondarily affected by infection are explored. Pulmonary vessels can spread infection to the lungs via septic emboli; alternatively, pulmonary vessels can be affected by infection in adjacent lung parenchyma acquired from the airways. Classic examples of acute bacterial infection, recurrent bacterial infection, septic embolism, and of mycobacterial, fungal, viral, and parasitic infections are used to illustrate the range of interplay between infections and pulmonary vessels.

◆ Acute Bacterial Infection

◆ Lobar consolidation can occur in acute bacterial pneumonia. On contrast material–enhanced computed tomography (CT), the contour of the vessels within areas of uncomplicated consolidation usually appears normal (**Fig. 8.1**).

◆ Local inflammation from lung infection leads to an increase in the production of tissue factor and the inhibition of fibrinolysis. In this procoagulant environment, focal in situ thrombosis can occasionally occur (see **Fig. 5.5** in Chapter 5).

◆ Consolidation causes a focal increase in pulmonary vascular resistance, which can slow the transit of blood and contrast material (see **Fig. 4.30** in Chapter 4). Unopacified blood can mimic pulmonary embolism or in situ thrombosis.

◆ Recurrent Bacterial Infection

◆ A pulmonary structural abnormality, such as the bronchiectasis seen in cystic fibrosis, can lead to recurrent bacterial infections.

◆ Recurrent infections in patients with cystic fibrosis can cause lung and vessel wall necrosis, characterized by

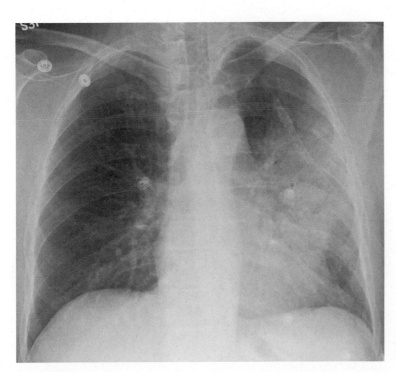

A

Fig. 8.1 (A–C) Acute streptococcal lobar pneumonia in a 54-year-old man. **(A)** Frontal chest radiograph demonstrates extensive consolidation with air bronchograms in the left lung. *(Continued on page 112)*

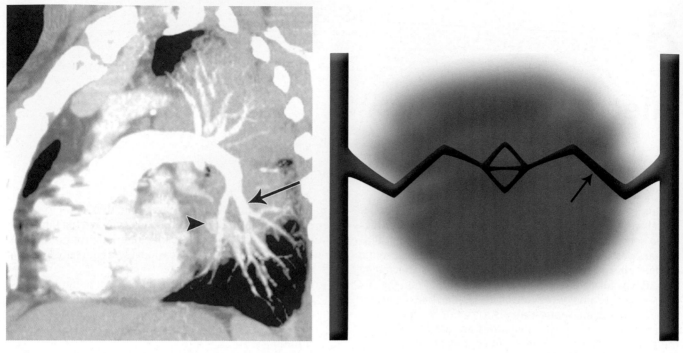

Fig. 8.1 (*Continued*) Acute streptococcal lobar pneumonia in a 54-year-old man. **(B)** Contrast material–enhanced CT maximum-intensity projection in a sagittal oblique plane demonstrates normal contours of the pulmonary arteries (*arrow*) and veins (*arrowhead*). **(C)** Illustration of pneumonia (represented by the *brown circle*). Coursing through the consolidated lung are vessels with normal contours and diameters (*arrow*).

hemorrhagic pneumonia, as well as bronchial artery and pulmonary artery pseudoaneurysm (**Fig. 8.2**).

♦ Massive hemoptysis in patients with cystic fibrosis is associated with *Staphylococcus aureus* infection and diabetes mellitus.

♦ Septic Emboli

♦ Septic emboli are seen in patients with infective endocarditis or periodontal disease. They are also associated with infected venous catheters or pacemaker leads.

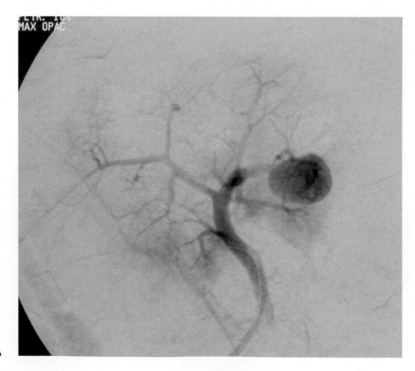

Fig. 8.2 **(A,B)** Pseudoaneurysm in a 25-year-old man with cystic fibrosis. **(A)** Spot film of a pulmonary angiogram demonstrates a pseudoaneurysm in the left upper lobe.

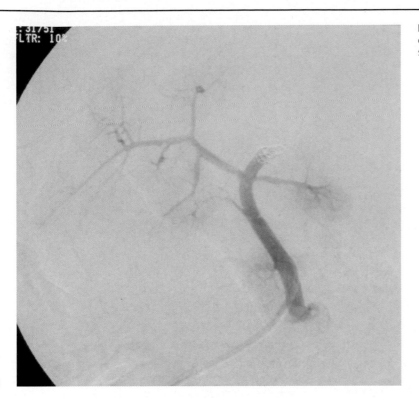

B

Fig. 8.2 (*Continued*) Pseudoaneurysm in a 25-year-old man with cystic fibrosis. **(B)** Spot film demonstrates successful coiling of the pseudoaneurysm.

- The infecting organism varies with the cause. In intravenous (I.V.) drug abusers, *S. aureus* is the most common infective agent.
- The radiologic appearances of septic emboli include nodules and wedge-shaped subpleural opacities with or without cavitation (**Fig. 8.3**).

◆ Mycobacterial Infection

- Tuberculous and nontuberculous mycobacteria often enter the lungs via the airways.
- Active primary or post-primary tuberculosis can affect the pulmonary vessels.

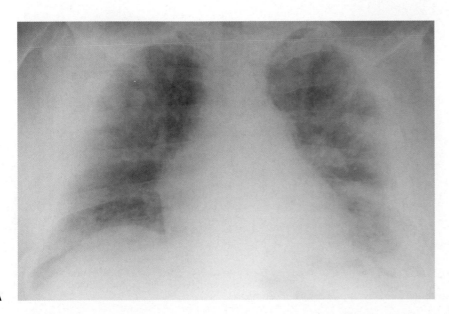

A

Fig. 8.3 **(A,B)** Septic emboli in a 28-year-old male I.V. drug abuser. **(A)** Frontal radiograph demonstrates bilateral, predominantly peripherally located ill-defined nodules. (*Continued on page 114*)

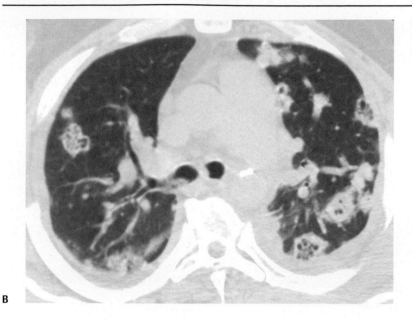

B

Fig. 8.3 (*Continued*) Septic emboli in a 28-year-old male I.V. drug abuser. **(B)** Corresponding CT demonstrates peripheral lobulated cavitary nodules in both lungs.

◆ Hemoptysis is a common presenting symptom and may be life-threatening.
◆ A necrotizing granulomatous pulmonary vasculitis can affect the pulmonary arteries and veins.
◆ The bronchial arteries are often enlarged in tuberculosis of the lung parenchyma; the source of hemoptysis in cavitary tuberculosis is usually the bronchial arteries (**Fig. 8.4**).

◆ Rasmussen aneurysm is a rare phenomenon caused by weakening of the pulmonary artery wall from adjacent cavitary tuberculosis (similar to **Fig. 8.2**).
◆ After entering the bloodstream, miliary tuberculosis of the lungs (**Fig. 8.5**) can spread via the bronchial and pulmonary arteries.

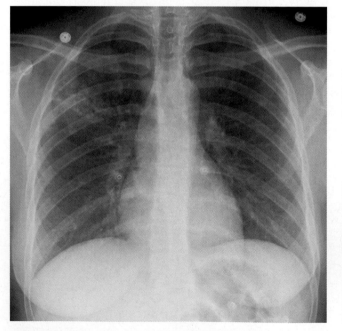

A

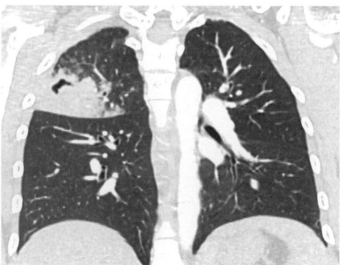

B

Fig. 8.4 (A–C) A 25-year-old woman with active tuberculosis and hemoptysis. **(A)** Chest radiograph demonstrates cavitary consolidation within the right upper lobe. **(B)** Coronal reconstruction CT shows the cavity more clearly. In addition, there are ill-defined nodules superior to the consolidation that could represent aspirated blood or tuberculous bronchopneumonia.

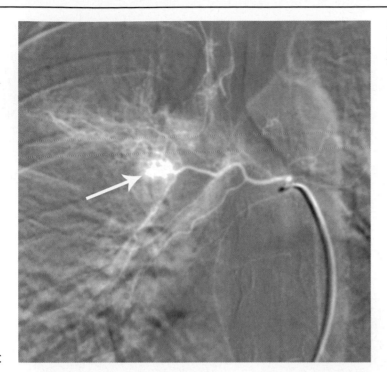

C

Fig. 8.4 (*Continued*) A 25-year-old woman with active tuberculosis and hemoptysis. **(C)** Bronchial angiogram demonstrates active hemorrhage from the bronchial artery supplying this infected region of the lung (*arrow*).

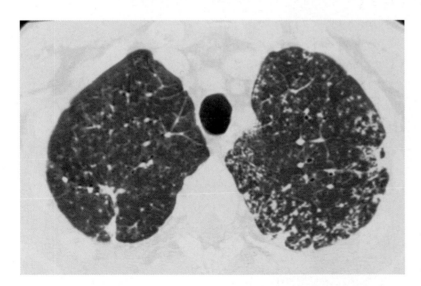

Fig. 8.5 Miliary tuberculosis in a 43-year-old man. High-resolution CT of the upper lobes demonstrates small nodules with a random distribution, a result of the hematogenous spread of miliary tuberculosis. Also seen are some branching tree-in-bud opacities in the left upper lobe, likely due to tuberculous bronchopneumonia.

◆ Fungal Infection

- ◆ Angio-invasive aspergillosis is used as an example of this group of diseases.
- ◆ This occurs almost exclusively in immunocompromised patients with severe neutropenia.
- ◆ It is characterized histologically by the invasion and occlusion of small to medium-size pulmonary arteries by fungal

hyphae, with the formation of necrotic hemorrhagic nodules or pleura-based, wedge-shaped hemorrhagic infarcts.
- ◆ The radiologic findings are nodules or masses (**Fig. 8.6**) surrounded by a halo of ground-glass attenuation or pleura-based, wedge-shaped areas of consolidation.
- ◆ Cavitation is usually seen during convalescence, 2 to 3 weeks after the initiation of treatment, and accompanies the resolution of neutropenia (**Fig. 8.6D**).

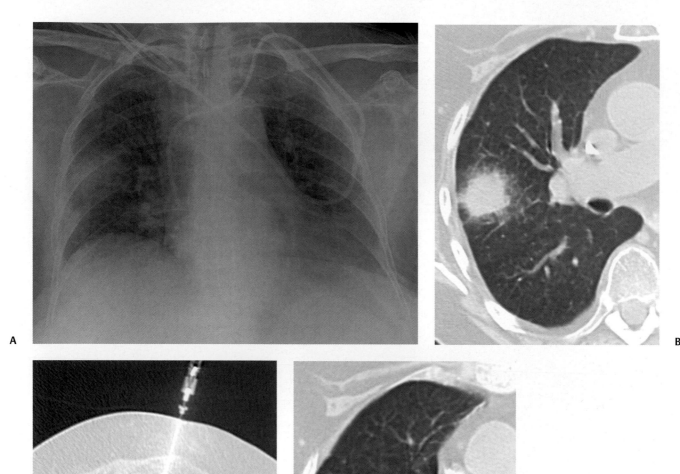

A

B

C

D

Fig. 8.6 (A–D) Angio-invasive aspergillosis in a 65-year-old woman. **(A)** Chest radiograph demonstrates a peripheral ill-defined mass in the right lung. **(B)** CT demonstrates a mass in the right upper lobe with a halo of ground-glass opacification, indicating pulmonary hemorrhage. **(C)** CT-guided lung biopsy demonstrates the needle tip in position, in the periphery of the lesion, before sampling of the lung mass. **(D)** After 2 weeks of therapy, CT demonstrates a slightly smaller lesion and classic cavitation within the mass.

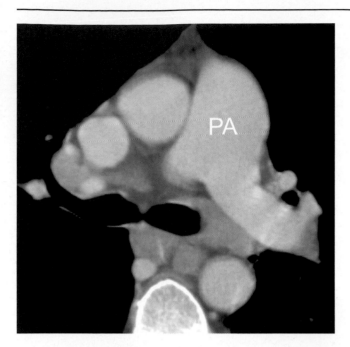

Fig. 8.7 Pulmonary artery hypertension in a 54-year-old man with HIV infection. CT demonstrates an enlarged main pulmonary artery (*PA*), consistent with pulmonary artery hypertension. Mediastinal lymphadenopathy is also present.

◆ Viral Infection

- Human immunodeficiency virus (HIV) infection is used as an example of this group of diseases.
- Interestingly, pulmonary arterial hypertension develops in 0.5% of patients with HIV infection (**Fig. 8.7**).
- The exact mechanism of development of HIV-related pulmonary hypertension is not clear. The predominant histopathologic finding is plexiform arteriopathy with adjacent perivascular inflammation.

- Bacillary angiomatosis is a manifestation of infection by *Bartonella henselae*, in which localized areas of vascular proliferation may affect the skin, airway, mucous membranes, visceral organs, bones, and brain.
- The mechanism of transmission is uncertain but is speculated to involve animals, including insect vectors.
- Bacillary angiomatosis occurs almost exclusively in patients with acquired immunodeficiency syndrome (AIDS).
- In the lung, this manifests radiographically as well- or ill-defined nodules (**Fig. 8.8**).

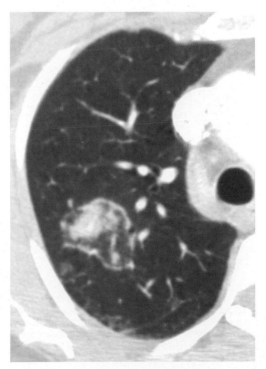

Fig. 8.8 Bacillary angiomatosis of the lung in a 47-year-old man. CT demonstrates an ill-defined nodule in the right upper lobe with some adjacent ground-glass opacification due to adjacent pulmonary hemorrhage.

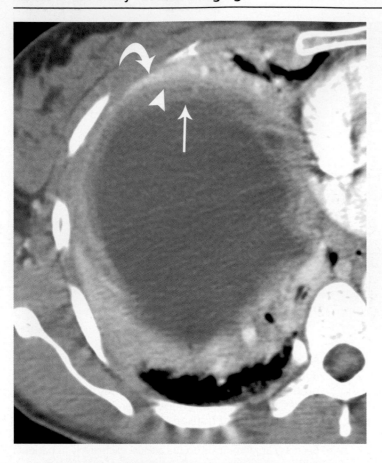

Fig. 8.9 Pulmonary hydatid disease in 25-year-old woman. CT demonstrates a large enhancing cystic mass within the right lower lobe. The thick wall consists of three layers: the endocyst (*arrow*), ectocyst (*arrowhead*), and pericyst (*curved arrow*).

◆ Parasitic Infection

◆ Parasites often spread to the lungs via the vasculature; pulmonary amebiasis and hydatid disease are examples (**Fig. 8.9**).

◆ Hydatid pulmonary artery embolism (**Fig. 8.10**) is a rare complication of cardiac or hepatic echinococcosis.

◆ Hydatid embolism can be acute and fatal, causing subacute pulmonary hypertension and death within 1 year after diagnosis, and is a cause of chronic pulmonary hypertension. In the majority of patients, the course of the disease consists of prolonged pulmonary hypertension punctuated by acute embolic episodes.

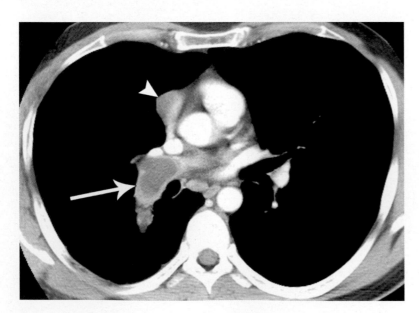

Fig. 8.10 Hydatid embolism in a 27-year-old man. CT demonstrates a well-enhanced branching hydatid embolism in the right lower and middle lobe pulmonary arteries (*arrow*); a small hydatid in the peripheral lung is also seen (*arrowhead*). (Courtesy of Dr. Federico Discepola.)

Suggested Reading

Dodd JD, Souza CA, Müller NL. High-resolution MDCT of pulmonary septic embolism: evaluation of the feeding vessel sign. AJR Am J Roentgenol 2006;187(3):623–629

Flume PA, Yankaskas JR, Ebeling M, Hulsey T, Clark LL. Massive hemoptysis in cystic fibrosis. Chest 2005;128(2):729–738

Franquet T, Müller NL, Giménez A, Guembe P, de La Torre J, Bagué S. Spectrum of pulmonary aspergillosis: histologic, clinical, and radiologic findings. Radiographics 2001;21(4):825–837

Han D, Lee KS, Franquet T, et al. Thrombotic and nonthrombotic pulmonary arterial embolism: spectrum of imaging findings. Radiographics 2003; 23(6):1521–1539

Kim HY, Song KS, Goo JM, Lee JS, Lee KS, Lim TH. Thoracic sequelae and complications of tuberculosis. Radiographics 2001;21(4):839–858, discussion 859–860

Moore EH, Russell LA, Klein JS, et al. Bacillary angiomatosis in patients with AIDS: multiorgan imaging findings. Radiology 1995;197(1):67–72

Shah RM, Friedman AC. CT angiogram sign: incidence and significance in lobar consolidations evaluated by contrast-enhanced CT. AJR Am J Roentgenol 1998;170(3):719–721

Sitbon O, Lascoux-Combe C, Delfraissy JF, et al. Prevalence of HIV-related pulmonary arterial hypertension in the current antiretroviral therapy era. Am J Respir Crit Care Med 2008;177(1):108–113

Tanoue LT, Mark EJ. Case records of the Massachusetts General Hospital. Weekly clinicopathological exercises. Case 1-2003. A 43-year-old man with fever and night sweats. N Engl J Med 2003;348(2):151–161

9

Trauma and Intervention

The pulmonary vessels can be injured by blunt or penetrating trauma directly, or they can be affected by trauma indirectly, as occurs with fat embolism. Pulmonary artery or vein transection and pseudoaneurysm are more common with penetrating trauma but can occur with blunt chest trauma. Peripheral interventions can affect the pulmonary vessels, most commonly with air embolism but also with catheter and cement embolism. Pulmonary vessel surgery or direct pulmonary vessel interventions can lead to in situ thrombosis, vessel stenosis, pseudoaneurysm and rupture, and occasionally fistula formation.

◆ Pseudoaneurysm

- ◆ A pseudoaneurysm, or false aneurysm, is one in which one or more of the arterial layers (adventitia, media, and intima) are missing.
- ◆ These tend to be saccular in shape (**Fig. 9.1**).

◆ Fat Embolism

- ◆ Fat embolism is an infrequent complication of fracture in a single long bone but is relatively common after more severe trauma. Other causes include hemoglobinopathies, major burns, pancreatitis, overwhelming infection, tumors, blood transfusion, and liposuction.
- ◆ The production of free fatty acids initiates a toxic reaction and inflammation centered on the endothelium. Also, fat globules and aggregates of red blood cells and platelets cause mechanical obstruction of the pulmonary vasculature.
- ◆ The classic clinical triad of hypoxia, neurologic abnormalities, and petechial rash occur within 12 to 24 hours after the traumatic event.
- ◆ Usually, 1 to 2 days elapse between the traumatic event and the appearance of radiographic abnormalities (see

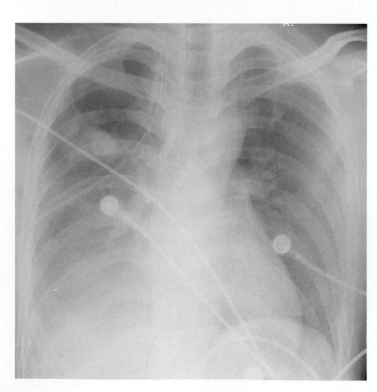

A

Fig. 9.1 (A–C) Pseudoaneurysm in a 23-year-old man with a stab wound. **(A)** Chest radiograph shows an ill-defined right upper lobe nodule, adjacent ground-glass opacification, and a moderate amount of right pleural fluid.

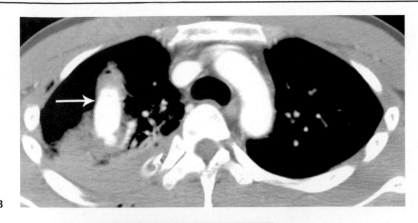

B

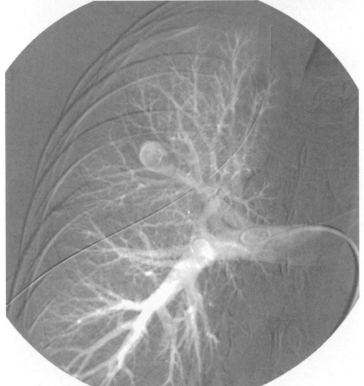

C

Fig. 9.1 (*Continued*) Pseudoaneurysm in a 23-year-old man with a stab wound. **(B)** Contrast material–enhanced CT demonstrates a large pseudoaneurysm in the right upper lobe (*arrow*) and adjacent pulmonary hemorrhage. **(C)** Right pulmonary angiogram before coiling confirms a pseudoaneurysm arising from the right upper lobe.

Fig. 4.42 in Chapter 4); this allows differentiation from traumatic contusion.

◆ Air Embolism

- Iatrogenic causes include injection of fluid including contrast material into venous catheters, transthoracic needle biopsy, and barotrauma resulting from positive-pressure ventilation.

- Air embolism occurs in up to 23% of patients given contrast material at computed tomography (CT; see **Fig. 4.37** in Chapter 4).
- Large volumes of air or right-to-left shunts can result in death or stroke.

◆ Catheter Embolism

- This iatrogenic embolism is due to catheter tear, which most often occurs on catheter removal (**Fig. 9.2**).

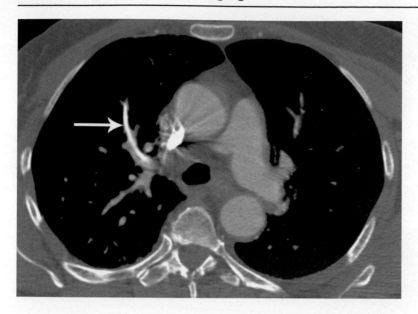

Fig. 9.2 Catheter embolism in a 59-year-old woman. CT demonstrates catheter within anterior segment of the right upper lobe pulmonary artery (*arrow*).

◆ Cement (Polymethylmethacrylate) Embolism

◆ The introduction of cement during percutaneous vertebroplasty is the most common cause of cement pulmonary embolism.

◆ Embolism is via the external vertebral venous plexuses to the pulmonary arteries (**Fig. 9.3**).

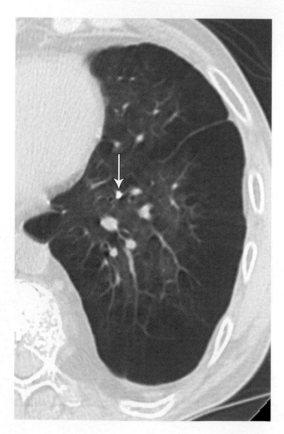

Fig. 9.3 Cement embolism in an 83-year-old man. CT demonstrates a subsegmental cement embolism within the left lower lobe (*arrow*).

◆ Pulmonary Artery Thrombosis

◆ Pulmonary artery stump thrombosis can be seen in 12% of patients who have undergone lung resection (see **Figs. 5.3** and **5.4** in Chapter 5).

◆ Nonobstructive pulmonary artery in situ thrombosis can occur in patients who have had a lung transplant (**Fig. 9.4**).

◆ Complete pulmonary artery obstruction after lung transplant has been seen in up to 4% of cases.

◆ Post–lung transplant pulmonary artery obstruction should be suspected in a patient with unexplained hypoxia or with new or recurrent pulmonary hypertension.

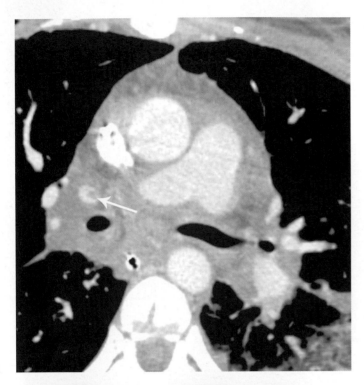

A

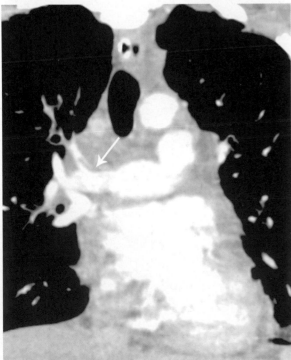

B

Fig. 9.4 (A,B) In situ pulmonary artery thrombosis in a 32-year-old woman after a right lobar transplant. **(A)** Axial CT demonstrates a nonobstructing in situ thrombus in the right upper pulmonary artery (*arrow*). **(B)** Coronal reconstruction CT also shows the in situ thrombus arising from the anastomotic site (*arrow*).

◆ Pulmonary Vein Thrombosis

- ◆ In situ thrombosis of the pulmonary vein has been described in patients who have undergone thoracic surgery for lobectomy or lung transplant or who have been treated with radio-frequency ablation. It is also seen in patients with chest trauma, left atrial dilatation, or atrial fibrillation.
- ◆ This is a potentially devastating disease that can lead to peripheral arterial embolism with transient ischemic attacks and stroke.
- ◆ Complete pulmonary vein obstruction after lung transplant has been seen in up to 1% of cases.
- ◆ Diagnostic tools include CT (see **Fig. 5.8** in Chapter 5), magnetic resonance imaging (MRI), and transesophageal echocardiography.

◆ Post-Lung Transplant Stenosis

- ◆ Vascular anastomotic stenosis or narrowing may occur as a consequence of donor-recipient size mismatch, surgical technique, or twisting. It may also occur after thrombosis of the pulmonary artery (**Figs. 9.5, 9.6,** and **9.7**).
- ◆ In severe cases, stenosis of the pulmonary artery or vein can have a significant hemodynamic effect, in which case stenting may be required.

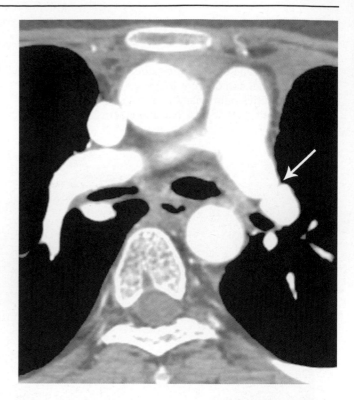

Fig. 9.5 Narrowing of a pulmonary artery anastomosis in a 24-year-old woman after a left lobar transplant. Contrast material–enhanced CT demonstrates minimal narrowing at the site of the anastomosis (*arrow*).

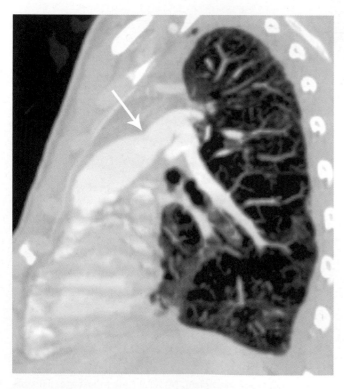

Fig. 9.6 Small-to-large vessel anastomosis in a 25-year-old man after a left lobar lung transplant. Contrast material–enhanced CT maximum-intensity projection (MIP) in the sagittal plane demonstrates anastomosis (*arrow*) of a small donor artery to a larger diameter native artery.

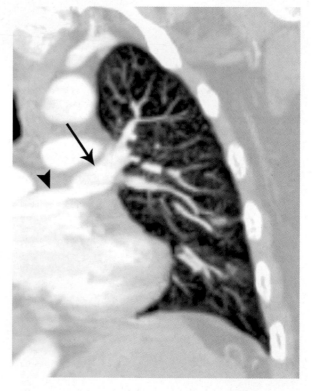

Fig. 9.7 Large-to-small vessel anastomosis in a 64-year-old man after a left lung transplant. Contrast material–enhanced CT MIP in the coronal plane demonstrates the anastomosis of a large transplant superior pulmonary vein (*arrow*) to a smaller native pulmonary vein (*arrowhead*).

◆ Pulmonary Vein Ablation Therapy

◆ Pulmonary vein ablation is a treatment option for paroxysmal atrial fibrillation.

◆ The energy required for this ablation procedure can come from several sources, including radio frequency and cord of cryotherapy.

◆ Pre-procedural examinations with CT or MRI are frequently performed to depict normal and variant anatomy and to obtain baseline measurements (**Fig. 9.8A**).

◆ Pulmonary vein stenosis (**Fig. 9.8B,C**), dissection, thrombosis, and infarction, as well as pulmonary hypertension and cardiac perforation, may all occur after ablation therapy.

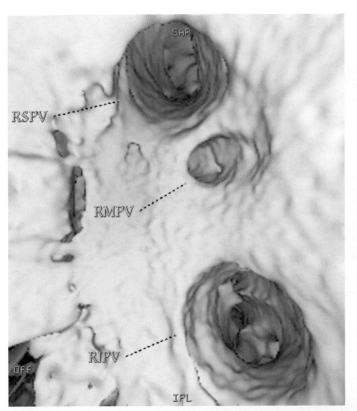

A

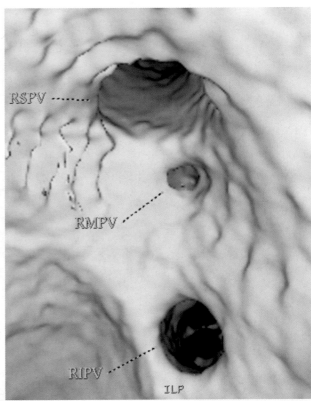

B

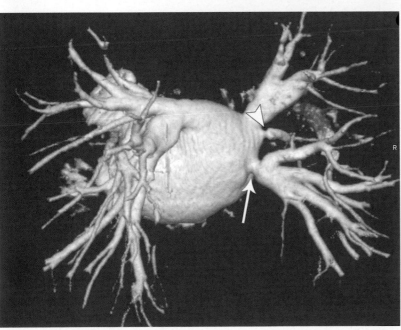

C

Fig. 9.8 (A–C) Pulmonary vein stenosis in a 58-year-old woman. **(A)** Before radio-frequency ablation, contrast material–enhanced three-dimensional surface-rendered MRI viewed from inside the left atrium demonstrates a normal-diameter right superior pulmonary vein (*RSPV*), right middle pulmonary vein (*RMPV*), and right inferior pulmonary vein (*RIPV*). **(B)** Pulmonary vein stenosis after radio-frequency ablation. In comparison with the image in **A**, the right middle pulmonary vein (*RMPV*) and right inferior pulmonary vein (*RIPV*) demonstrate significant narrowing. *RSPV*, right superior pulmonary vein. **(C)** Contrast material–enhanced three-dimensional surface-rendered MRI viewed from outside the left atrium demonstrates approximately 50% stenosis of the right middle pulmonary vein (*arrowhead*) and right inferior pulmonary vein (*arrow*).

◆ Pulmonary Artery Catheter Injury

- ◆ This iatrogenic injury is due to malposition of the pulmonary artery catheter, in which the tip location is often too peripheral.

- ◆ The catheter tip can erode the artery wall, resulting in a pseudoaneurysm that is often saccular (**Fig. 9.9**).
- ◆ The incidence of rupture resulting from insertion of a pulmonary artery catheter is estimated at 0.03%; the mortality rate after rupture is 70% (**Fig. 9.10**).

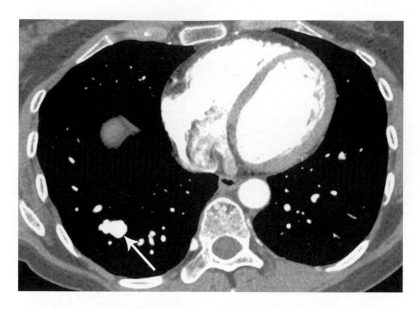

Fig. 9.9 Pulmonary artery pseudoaneurysm in a 48-year-old man after pulmonary artery catheterization. CT demonstrates a lobulated saccular aneurysm within the right lower lobe (*arrow*).

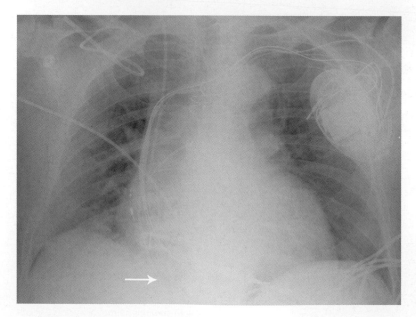

A

Fig. 9.10 (A,B) Massive hemoptysis in a 78-year-old man after insertion of a pulmonary artery line. **(A)** The chest radiograph demonstrates the tip of the pulmonary artery line in one of the subsegmental arteries of the right lower lobe (*arrow*) just before massive hemoptysis and right-sided thoracotomy and repair.

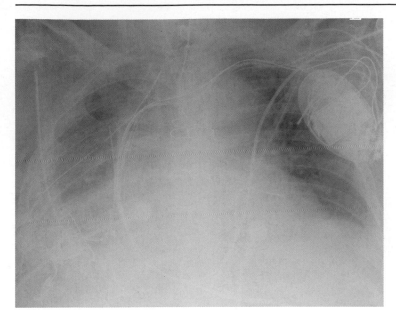

Fig. 9.10 (*Continued*) Massive hemoptysis in a 78-year-old man after insertion of a pulmonary artery line. **(B)** Immediately after right lower lobe pulmonary artery repair, chest radiograph demonstrates numerous right-sided chest drains and right lower lobe consolidation, consistent with hemorrhage or postoperative contusion.

B

◆ Fistula

◆ A fistula is an abnormal connection between an organ (e.g., the intestine) or vessel and another structure.

◆ Trauma or interventions can lead to abnormal communications between vessels, including pulmonary arteriovenous fistulas and systemic-to-pulmonary vessel shunts (**Fig. 9.11**).

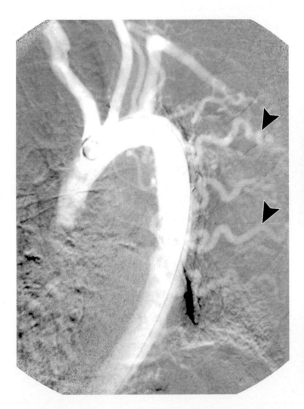

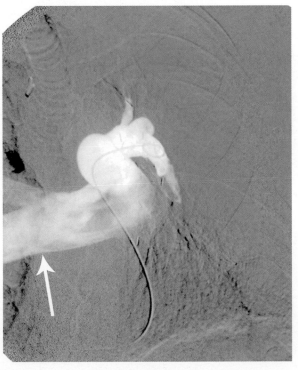

A B

Fig. 9.11 (A,B) Systemic-to-pulmonary artery shunt in a 59-year-old man after left upper lobectomy and lung volume reduction surgery. **(A)** Arch aortogram demonstrates numerous dilated collateral intercostal arteries (*arrowheads*). **(B)** In a left pulmonary artery arteriogram, blood is seen to cross over from the left to the right pulmonary artery (*arrow*), indicating higher systemic pressure in the left pulmonary artery.

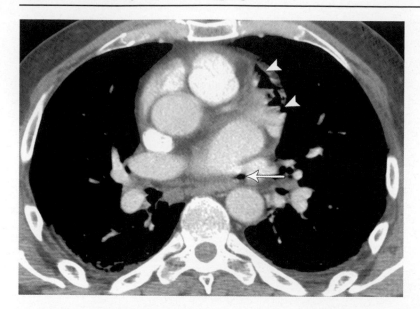

Fig. 9.12 Fistula from pulmonary vein to esophagus in a 56-year-old man who had a stroke after radio-frequency ablation therapy of the pulmonary veins. CT demonstrates a small fleck of air (*arrow*) at the site of the fistula and air within the left atrial appendage (*arrowheads*).

◆ Trauma or interventions can also lead to abnormal communications between vessels and the gastrointestinal tract. Within the thorax, such communications are generally with the esophagus (**Fig. 9.12**).

Suggested Reading

Clark SC, Levine AJ, Hasan A, Hilton CJ, Forty J, Dark JH. Vascular complications of lung transplantation. Ann Thorac Surg 1996;61(4):1079–1082

Ghaye B, Szapiro D, Dacher JN, et al. Percutaneous ablation for atrial fibrillation: the role of cross-sectional imaging. Radiographics 2003; 23(Spec No):S19–S33, discussion S48–S50

Gill RR, Poh AC, Camp PC, et al. MDCT evaluation of central airway and vascular complications of lung transplantation. AJR Am J Roentgenol 2008;191(4):1046–1056

Kearney TJ, Shabot MM. Pulmonary artery rupture associated with the Swan-Ganz catheter. Chest 1995;108(5):1349–1352

Pereira SJ, Narrod JA. Repair of right pulmonary artery transection after blunt trauma. Ann Thorac Surg 2009;87(3):939–940

Symbas PN, Goldman M, Erbesfeld MH, Vlasis SE. Pulmonary arteriovenous fistula, pulmonary artery aneurysm, and other vascular changes of the lung from penetrating trauma. Ann Surg 1980;191(3):336–340

Weltman DI, Baykal A, Zhang D. CT diagnosis of laceration of the main pulmonary artery after blunt trauma. AJR Am J Roentgenol 1999; 173(5):1361–1362

10

Tumor

The majority of primary pulmonary vascular tumors are sarcomas that most often arise in the large pulmonary arteries and less commonly the pulmonary veins. More peripherally located primary vascular neoplasms include Kaposi sarcoma, intravascular lymphoma, and epithelioid hemangioendothelioma. Secondary involvement of the pulmonary vasculature by lung metastatic deposits may mimic primary vascular tumors, and multifocal micrometastases can cause unexplained pulmonary arterial hypertension. Primary bronchogenic neoplasia may locally invade, and on occasion obliterate, pulmonary arteries and veins. This chapter also illustrates how the treatment of lung cancer can affect the pulmonary vasculature.

◆ Primary Sarcoma

- ◆ Primary sarcoma is an uncommon cause of an intraluminal filling defect in a pulmonary vessel.
- ◆ Undifferentiated sarcoma and leiomyosarcoma are the most frequent histologic types that affect large pulmonary vessels, more often the arteries than the veins.
- ◆ A primary sarcoma manifests as a lobulated, heterogeneously enhancing mass on computed tomography (CT; **Fig. 10.1**) or magnetic resonance imaging (MRI) and can occasionally demonstrate calcifications on non–contrast-enhanced CT (**Fig. 10.2**).
- ◆ It often demonstrates vascular distension and local extravascular extension (**Figs. 10.1** and **10.2**).

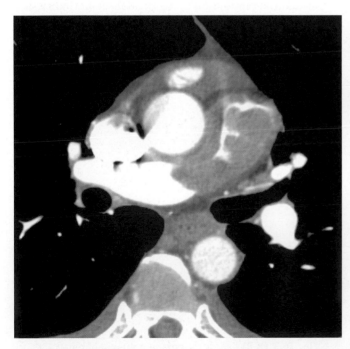

A

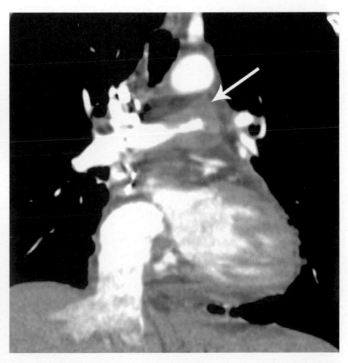

B

Fig. 10.1 (A,B) Pulmonary artery sarcoma in a 52-year-old man. **(A)** CT demonstrates a lobulated long mass extending from the main to the right pulmonary artery. **(B)** Coronal reconstruction CT demonstrates that the mass extends beyond the superior boundary of the pulmonary artery (*arrow*), indicating local invasion by a malignancy.

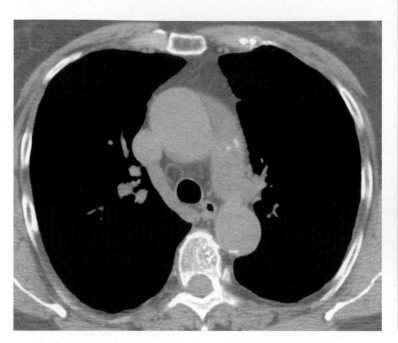

A

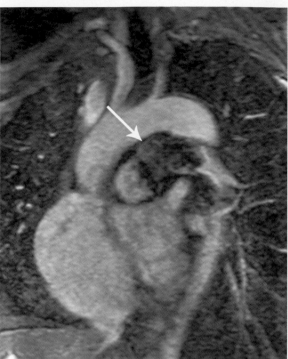

B

Fig. 10.2 (A,B) Pulmonary artery sarcoma in a 75-year-old woman. **(A)** Unenhanced CT demonstrates the hint of a mass and calcification within the main and left pulmonary arteries. **(B)** Coronal oblique contrast material–enhanced MRI demonstrates the enhancing tumor invading locally beyond the superior vessel wall (*arrow*).

◆ Kaposi Sarcoma

- ◆ Kaposi sarcoma is the most common tumor among patients with human immunodeficiency virus (HIV) infection and is associated with human herpesvirus 8 infection.
- ◆ Despite its name, it is not a true sarcoma (which normally arises from mesenchymal tissue). Kaposi sarcoma is a cancer of the lymphatic and blood endothelium that forms vascular channels that fill with blood.
- ◆ Highly active antiretroviral therapy has resulted in a substantial diminution in the incidence, morbidity, and mortality of Kaposi sarcoma. However, the radiologic appearance has remained similar (**Fig. 10.3**).

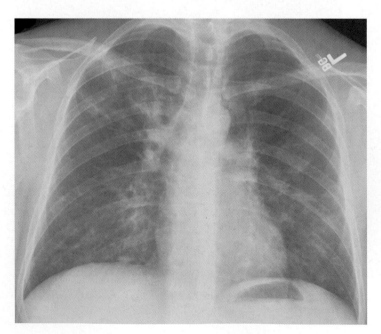

A

Fig. 10.3 (A,B) Kaposi sarcoma in a 40-year-old man with acquired immunodeficiency syndrome (AIDS). **(A)** Posteroanterior radiograph demonstrates bilateral ill-defined nodular opacities and reticular opacities, particularly of the lower lobes.

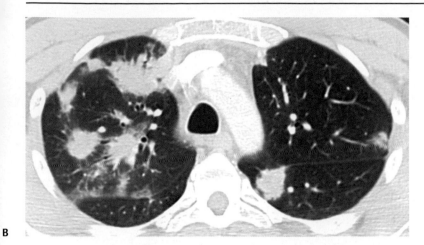

Fig. 10.3 (*Continued*) Kaposi sarcoma in a 40-year-old man with acquired immunodeficiency syndrome (AIDS). **(B)** CT demonstrates irregular nodules and masses with a predominantly peribronchovascular distribution.

B

◆ Intravascular Lymphoma

◆ Intravascular lymphoma is a very uncommon non-Hodgkin lymphoma characterized by the neoplastic proliferation of lymphoid cells within the lumina of capillaries, small veins, and arteries, with little or no adjacent parenchymal involvement.

◆ The CT finding is a ground-glass opacity containing small linear and nodular opacities in the affected lung (**Fig. 10.4**).

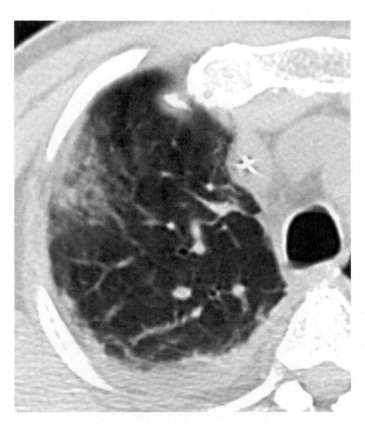

Fig. 10.4 Intravascular lymphoma in a 61-year-old man. CT demonstrates a peripheral ground-glass opacity containing small linear and nodular opacities within the right upper lobe. There is also a small right pleural effusion.

◆ Epithelioid Hemangioendothelioma

- ◆ Epithelioid hemangioendothelioma is a low-grade vascular tumor that most often primarily affects the lung or liver.
- ◆ The tumor may originate in either organ and metastasize to the other.
- ◆ The CT findings include bilateral lung nodules surrounded by ground-glass opacification suggesting pulmonary hemorrhage (**Fig. 10.5**).

◆ Metastatic Vascular Tumors

- ◆ Angiosarcomas are uncommon malignant vascular tumors associated with a high rate of metastatic involvement of the lungs.
- ◆ Patients present with dyspnea, chest pain, and/or hemoptysis.
- ◆ The most common radiologic findings are lung nodules (**Fig. 10.6**).

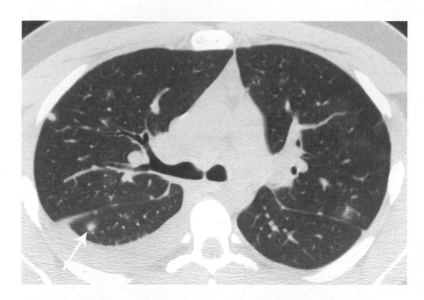

Fig. 10.5 Epithelioid hemangioendothelioma in a 20-year-old man with back pain and hemoptysis. CT demonstrates lung nodules with a ground-glass halo (*arrow*). There is also a small right pleural effusion.

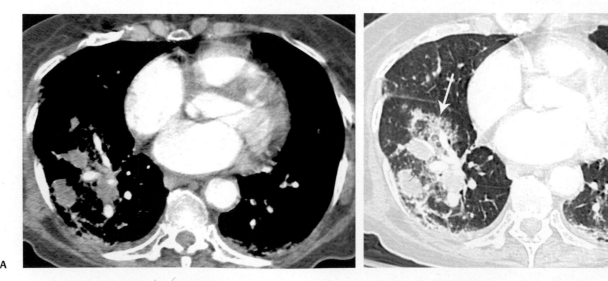

A

B

Fig. 10.6 (A,B) Metastatic angiosarcoma in an 83-year-old man with hemoptysis. **(A)** CT demonstrates enhancing masses within the right lower lobe. **(B)** On lung window settings, there is peritumoral ground-glass opacification (*arrow*), consistent with pulmonary hemorrhage.

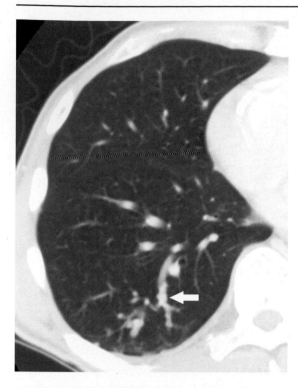

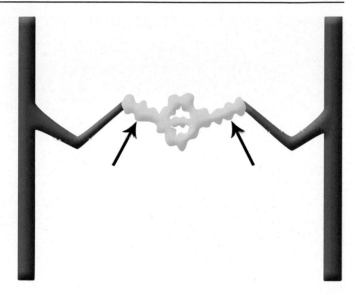

Fig. 10.8 Illustration of the effect of tumor on pulmonary vessels. Microembolism of tumor (represented by *yellow lobulated abnormality* in capillaries) can cause expansion of the vessels and grows along afferent and efferent vessel lumina (*arrows*).

Fig. 10.7 Tumor embolism in a 60-year-old man with dyspnea and primary renal cell carcinoma. CT scan shows tumor emboli that manifest as vascular dilatation and beading of subsegmental arteries of the posterobasal segment of the right pulmonary artery (*arrow*).

◆ Tumor Embolism

- ◆ Multifocal micrometastatic tumor emboli associated with dyspnea are found most commonly in patients with carcinomas of the breast, lung, stomach, or prostate gland.
- ◆ Tumor emboli that affect subsegmental arteries can produce vascular dilatation and beading that, without treatment, increase in size over time (**Figs. 10.7** and **10.8**).
- ◆ Small tumor emboli can affect secondary pulmonary lobule arterioles and have a centrilobular nodule or tree-in-bud appearance (**Fig. 10.8**; see also **Fig. 4.44** in Chapter 4).

◆ Lung Cancer

- ◆ Non–small-cell lung cancers that invade the great vessels and/or heart are T4 tumors in the tumor-node-metastasis (TNM) classification and have generally been considered

inoperable. However, the indication for the surgical resection of lung cancers has recently been expanded to include some patients with T4 disease.
- ◆ Accurate evaluation is vital for adequate surgical planning because the surgical manipulation of lung cancer within the pulmonary veins or left atrium may result in systemic tumor embolization.
- ◆ Lung cancer, by mass effect, can compress the pulmonary vessels (**Figs. 10.9** and **10.10**).
- ◆ A tumor can invade and grow along pulmonary vessels farther than it can along its lung interface (**Figs. 10.11, 10.12,** and **10.13**).
- ◆ It can completely obliterate the affected vessel (**Figs. 10.14** and **10.15**).

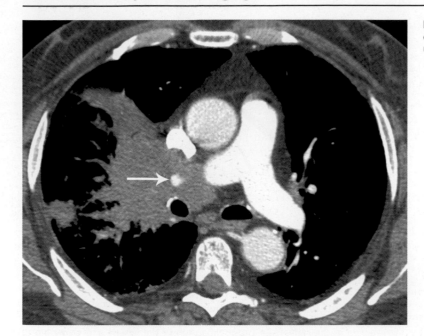

Fig. 10.9 Primary lung cancer in a 74-year-old man. CT demonstrates compression and narrowing of the right upper lobe pulmonary artery (*arrow*).

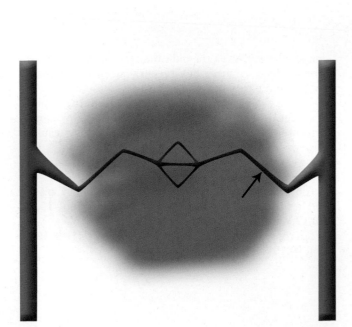

Fig. 10.10 Illustration of the effect of tumor on pulmonary vessels. The tumor (represented by *brown circle*) can cause a mass effect and compression of the pulmonary vessels (*arrow*).

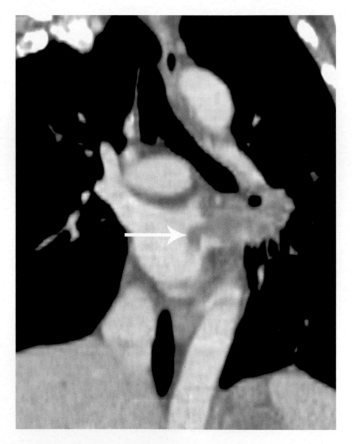

Fig. 10.11 Primary lung cancer in a 73-year-old man. Coronal reconstruction CT demonstrates a mass invading the left inferior pulmonary vein and a component within the left atrium (*arrow*).

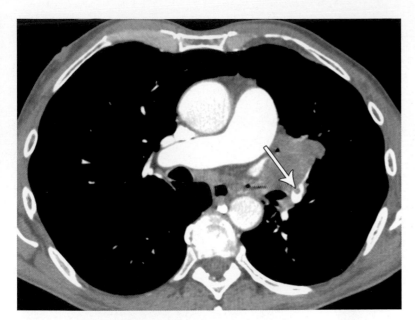

Fig. 10.12 Pulmonary artery tumor invasion in a 65-year-old man. CT demonstrates a large adenocarcinoma in the hilum of the left lung with direct local invasion of the left lower lobe pulmonary artery (*arrow*).

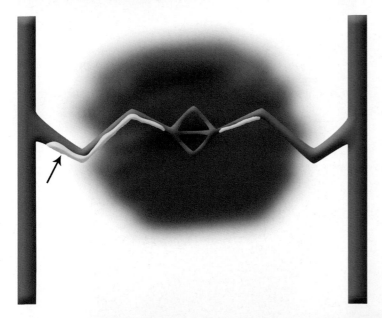

Fig. 10.13 Illustration of the effect of tumor on pulmonary vessels. The primary tumor (represented by *brown circle*) can invade pulmonary arteries and veins (represented by *yellow abnormality* in vessels). The vessel can serve as a route for local metastatic spread (*arrow*) beyond the edge of the primary neoplasm.

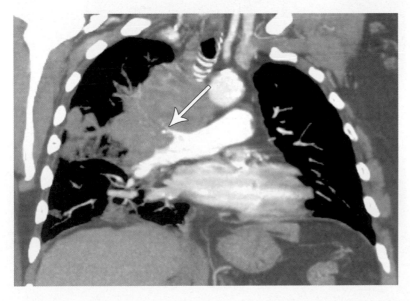

Fig. 10.14 Primary lung cancer in a 74-year-old man. Coronal reconstruction CT demonstrates complete obliteration of the right upper lobe pulmonary artery (*arrow*).

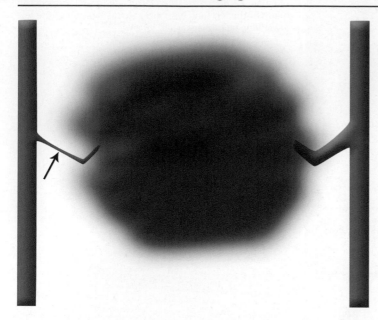

Fig. 10.15 Illustration of the effect of tumor on pulmonary vessels. The primary lung neoplasm (represented by *brown circle*) can obliterate pulmonary vessels within the mass. The efferent pulmonary veins also become narrowed because of a lack of blood flow (*arrow*).

◆ Radiotherapy

◆ The late effects of radiation are due to the proliferation of endothelial and smooth-muscle cells and to perivascular fibrosis, which can result in vessel lumen narrowing (**Fig. 10.16**) and complete obliteration.

◆ Chemotherapy can exacerbate this iatrogenic vascular injury.

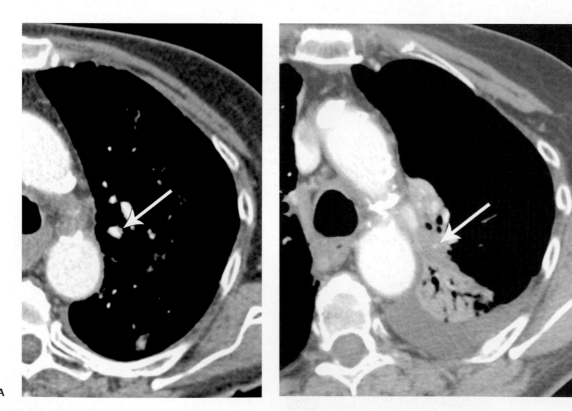

Fig. 10.16 (A,B) A 79-year-old women with lung cancer. **(A)** Before radiotherapy, CT demonstrates a normal-caliber left upper lobe posterior pulmonary artery (*arrow*). **(B)** Ten months after radiotherapy, the same artery is significantly reduced in diameter because of fibrosis (*arrow*).

Suggested Reading

Bocklage T, Leslie K, Yousem S, Colby T. Extracutaneous angiosarcomas metastatic to the lungs: clinical and pathologic features of twenty-one cases. Mod Pathol 2001;14(12):1216–1225

Burke AP, Virmani R. Sarcomas of the great vessels. A clinicopathologic study. Cancer 1993;71(5):1761–1773

Cox JE, Chiles C, Aquino SL, Savage P, Oaks T. Pulmonary artery sarcomas: a review of clinical and radiologic features. J Comput Assist Tomogr 1997;21(5):750–755

Demirer T, Dail DH, Aboulafia DM. Four varied cases of intravascular lymphomatosis and a literature review. Cancer 1994;73(6):1738–1745

Gladish GW, Sabloff BM, Munden RF, Truong MT, Erasmus JJ, Chasen MH. Primary thoracic sarcomas. Radiographics 2002;22(3):621–637

Godoy MC, Rouse H, Brown JA, Phillips P, Forrest DM, Müller NL. Imaging features of pulmonary Kaposi sarcoma-associated immune reconstitution syndrome. AJR Am J Roentgenol 2007;189(4): 956–965

Kane RD, Hawkins HK, Miller JA, Noce PS. Microscopic pulmonary tumor emboli associated with dyspnea. Cancer 1975;36(4): 1473–1482

Kradin RL, Mark EJ. Case Records of the Massachusetts General Hospital. Weekly clinicopathological exercises. Case 6-2000. Hemoptysis in a 20-year-old man with multiple pulmonary nodules. N Engl J Med 2000;342(8):572–578

Piedbois P, Becquemin JP, Blanc I, et al. Arterial occlusive disease after radiotherapy: a report of fourteen cases. Radiother Oncol 1990;17(2): 133–140

Tack D, Nollevaux MC, Gevenois PA. Tree-in-bud pattern in neoplastic pulmonary emboli. AJR Am J Roentgenol 2001;176(6):1421–1422

Takahashi K, Furuse M, Hanaoka H, et al. Pulmonary vein and left atrial invasion by lung cancer: assessment by breath-hold gadolinium-enhanced three-dimensional MR angiography. J Comput Assist Tomogr 2000;24(4):557–561

Wittram C, Maher MM, Yoo AJ, Kalra MK, Shepard JA, McLoud TC. CT angiography of pulmonary embolism: diagnostic criteria and causes of misdiagnosis. Radiographics 2004;24(5):1219–1238

Yi CA, Lee KS, Choe YH, Han D, Kwon OJ, Kim S. Computed tomography in pulmonary artery sarcoma: distinguishing features from pulmonary embolic disease. J Comput Assist Tomogr 2004;28(1):34–39

Yi ES. Tumors of the pulmonary vasculature. Cardiol Clin 2004;22(3): 431–440, vi–vii

11

Systemic and Lung Diseases

In this chapter, examples are used to illustrate how certain systemic and lung diseases, not already covered in previous chapters, can manifest and affect the appearance of the pulmonary vasculature. The diseases explored here include sarcoidosis, hepatopulmonary syndrome, sickle cell disease, bronchopulmonary dysplasia, idiopathic pulmonary hemosiderosis, emphysema, pulmonary Langerhans cell histiocytosis, usual interstitial pneumonitis, lymphangiomatosis and the angiomatous diseases, which include capillary hemangiomatosis and pulmonary capillary veno-occlusive disease.

◆ Sarcoidosis

◆ Sarcoidosis is a systemic noncaseating granulomatous disease of unknown etiology that affects the mediastinum, lungs, and other organs to varying degrees.
◆ In its most severe form, sarcoidosis can manifest as fibrosing mediastinitis with obliteration of the pulmonary arteries (**Fig. 11.1**) and veins (**Fig. 11.2**).

◆ Pulmonary hypertension occurs in patients with end-stage lung disease due to sarcoidosis; several mechanisms may contribute, including fibrotic destruction of the capillary bed and resultant chronic hypoxemia, extrinsic compression of the major pulmonary arteries by enlarged lymph nodes, and secondary pulmonary veno-occlusive disease.

◆ Hepatopulmonary Syndrome

◆ Hepatopulmonary syndrome is defined as the triad of hepatic dysfunction, intrapulmonary vascular dilatation, and hypoxemia.
◆ Clinically, it manifests as progressive dyspnea in patients with cirrhosis.
◆ It occurs in 50% of patients with chronic liver disease of any cause.
◆ It is not to be confused with portopulmonary hypertension, which is pulmonary hypertension due to increased vascular resistance in patients with portal hypertension.

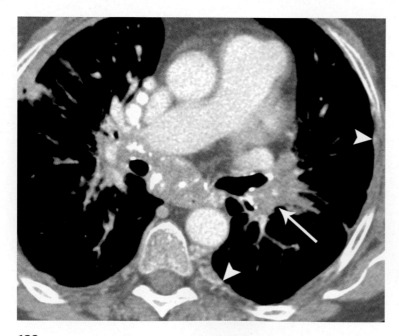

Fig. 11.1 Fibrosing mediastinitis due to sarcoidosis in a 72-year-old man. Axial CT demonstrates extensive mediastinal and hilar lymphadenopathy. There is obliteration of the left lower lobe pulmonary artery by the fibrotic mass (*arrow*) and intercostal artery collaterals (*arrowheads*).

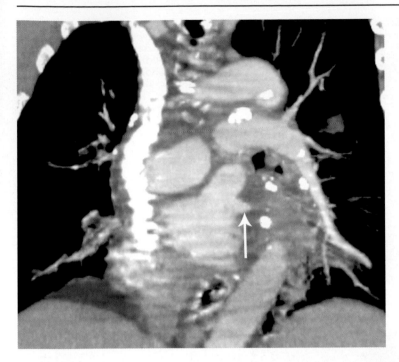

Fig. 11.2 Fibrosing mediastinitis due to sarcoidosis in a 61-year-old man. Coronal reconstruction CT demonstrates obliteration of the left inferior pulmonary vein (*arrow*) secondary to sarcoidosis.

◆ Normal pulmonary capillaries are between 8 and 15 μm in diameter; in hepatopulmonary syndrome, they are 15 to 100 μm in diameter.

◆ The hypoxemia is due to the presence of numerous tiny intrapulmonary shunts.

◆ Radiographic findings include bilateral basilar nodular or reticular opacities on chest radiograph, heterogeneous uptake on perfusion lung scan, and peripheral arteriolar dilatation on computed tomography (CT) or magnetic resonance imaging (MRI; **Fig. 11.3**).

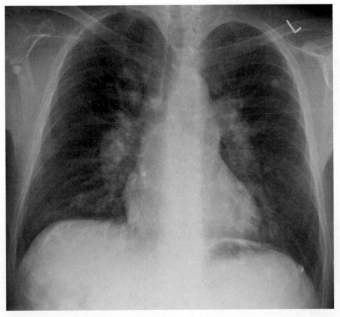

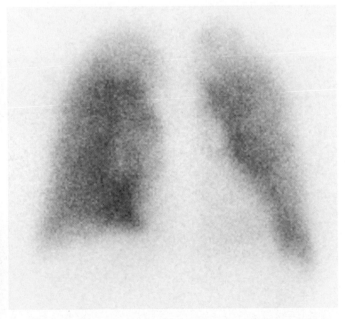

A

B

Fig. 11.3 (A–E) Hepatopulmonary syndrome in a 47-year-old man. **(A)** Chest radiograph demonstrates a heart of normal size with dilated central and peripheral pulmonary arteries. **(B)** Technetium Tc 99m macroaggregate (^{99m}Tc-macroaggregate) albumin perfusion scan demonstrates heterogeneous pulmonary perfusion with no segmental defects. The ventilation scan result was normal. (*Continued on page 140*)

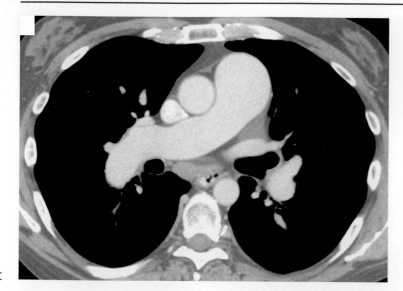

C

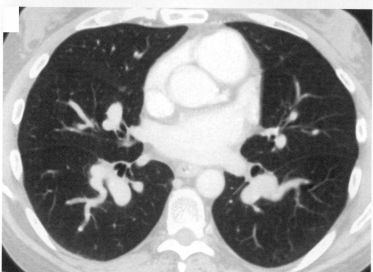

D

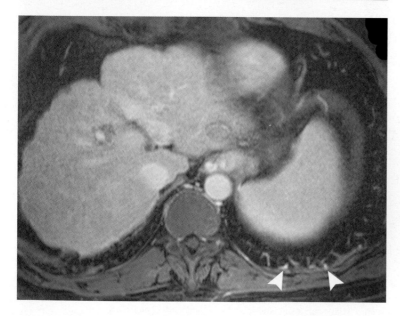

E

Fig. 11.3 (*Continued*) Hepatopulmonary syndrome in a 47-year-old man. **(C)** CT demonstrates dilated main, right, and left pulmonary arteries. **(D)** CT demonstrates dilated segmental arteries (the diameter of the artery is much larger than the diameter of the accompanying bronchus); also, there are dilated and tortuous subsegmental arteries. **(E)** MRI shows dilated subpleural pulmonary vessels (*arrowheads*). In addition, a small nodular liver and esophageal varices are seen.

◆ Sickle Cell Disease

◆ Sickle cell disease is a systemic disease that can result in occlusion of the small pulmonary vessels.

◆ In the acute chest syndrome, capillary obstruction by sickle cells is accompanied by in situ thrombosis.

◆ Imaging can demonstrate ground-glass opacification or extensive consolidation due to hemorrhagic edema, which is caused by ischemia, infarction, or infection and is responsible for precipitation of the acute chest syndrome (**Fig. 11.4**).

◆ CT can show mosaic attenuation, thought to be related to secondary pulmonary lobules with hypoperfusion adjacent to normal or hyperperfused lobules (**Fig. 11.4**).

◆ Chronic changes are seen in individuals experiencing repeated acute episodes, with parenchymal bands due to fibrosis of infarctions (**Fig. 11.4**).

◆ Eventually, in patients with persistent occlusion of the microvascular bed, cor pulmonale develops, manifested as dilatation of the pulmonary arteries and right ventricular hypertrophy.

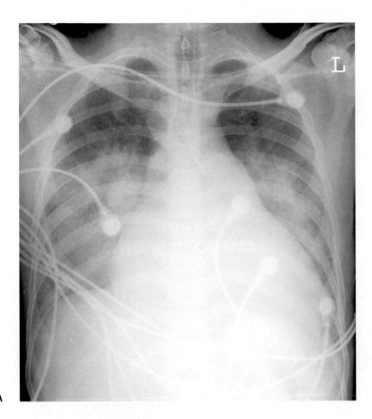

A

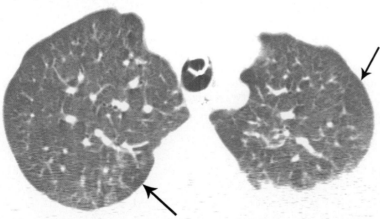

B

Fig. 11.4 (A–D) Sickle cell crisis in a 27-year-old man. **(A)** Chest radiograph demonstrates that the patient is intubated. Even allowing for the projection, the heart appears enlarged and the main pulmonary artery prominent. There is bilateral consolidation, which can represent pulmonary infarction or precipitating pneumonia. **(B)** CT performed at the same time as chest radiography demonstrates bilateral upper lobe mosaic attenuation. The more lucent regions represent poorly perfused lobules (*arrows*). (*Continued on page 142*)

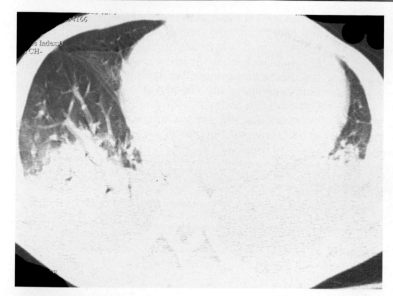

C

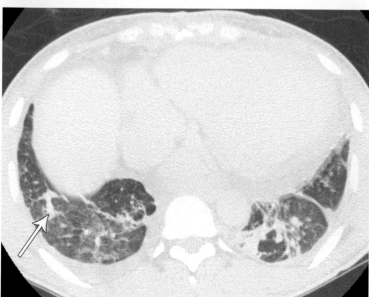

D

Fig. 11.4 (*Continued*) Sickle cell crisis in a 27-year-old man. **(C)** More inferiorly, CT demonstrates bilateral lower lobe consolidation. **(D)** CT performed at a later date demonstrates bilateral linear lung scars, manifested as bands (*arrow*), as well as a persistent mosaic pattern of lung attenuation.

◆ Bronchopulmonary Dysplasia

◆ In premature neonates, the high pressures of oxygen delivery can result in necrotizing vasculitis, bronchiolitis, and alveolar septal injury.

◆ CT features in older survivors include extensive areas of decreased lung attenuation, within which the size and number of vessels and bronchi are reduced as a consequence of chronic changes in the lung parenchyma, vessels, and airways (**Fig. 11.5**).

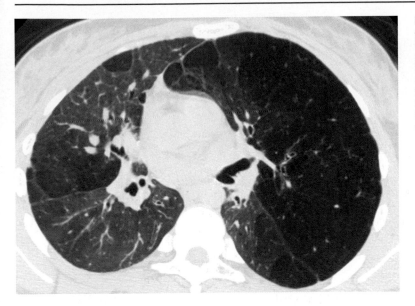

Fig. 11.5 Bronchopulmonary dysplasia in a 13-year-old girl. High-resolution CT demonstrates a mosaic pattern of lung attenuation. The more lucent regions of lung have small vessels, consistent with chronic vessel damage or shunting of blood to the more attenuating and functional regions of lung. There is also shift of the mediastinum from left to right secondary to a large left lung volume resulting from air trapping. The bronchi and bronchioles in the lucent regions of lung are also noted to be small in diameter.

◆ Idiopathic Pulmonary Hemosiderosis

- Idiopathic pulmonary hemosiderosis is a rare cause of diffuse alveolar hemorrhage and, by definition, of unknown etiology.
- The cause is thought to be a defect in the alveolar basement membrane.
- It occurs most frequently in children, has a variable natural history with repetitive episodes of diffuse alveolar hemorrhage, and can be fatal.

- Iron deficiency anemia develops in many cases.
- Sputum and bronchoalveolar lavage fluid can disclose hemosiderin-laden alveolar macrophages, and lung biopsy shows similar findings in the alveoli, without evidence of pulmonary vasculitis, granulomatous inflammation, or immunoglobulin deposition.
- Imaging studies often show diffuse ground-glass opacification and, later in the course of the disease, minimal interstitial fibrosis (**Fig. 11.6**).

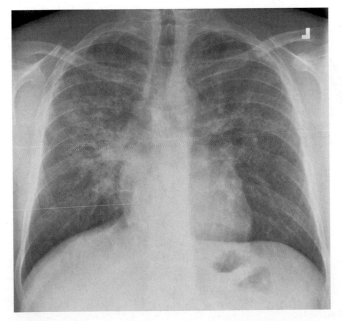

A

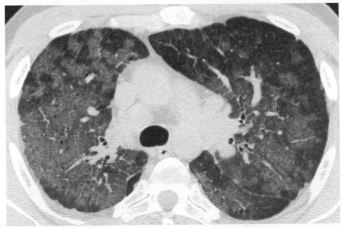

B

Fig. 11.6 (A–C) Hemosiderosis in a 23-year-old man. **(A)** Chest radiograph demonstrates a diffuse increase in the attenuation of the lungs and almost consolidation adjacent to the right hilum inferiorly.

(B) High-resolution CT shows diffuse ground-glass opacity. (*Continued on page 144*)

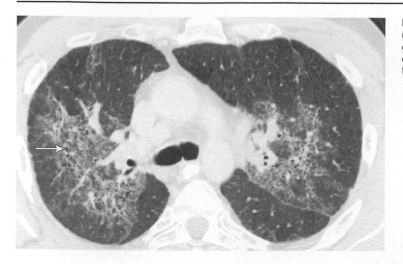

Fig. 11.6 (*Continued*) Hemosiderosis in a 23-year-old man. **(C)** High-resolution CT more inferiorly shows perihilar ground-glass opacities and fine reticulation, as well as distortion of the oblique fissures and bronchial dilatation (*arrow*), indicative of fibrosis.

C

◆ Emphysema

- ◆ Centrilobular emphysema due to cigarette smoking classically affects the upper lobes most severely.
- ◆ Pulmonary arteriolar constriction in response to local hypoxia reduces perfusion in poorly ventilated or non-ventilated lung units in the upper lobes, and blood is diverted to better-ventilated lung units in the lower lobes (**Fig. 11.7**).
- ◆ Pulmonary hypertension develops as a consequence of chronic hypoxia as well as the pathologic conditions affecting the vessels: intimal thickening, muscularization of arterioles, in situ thrombosis, loss of capillaries and precapillary arterioles, and vascular congestion and stasis.

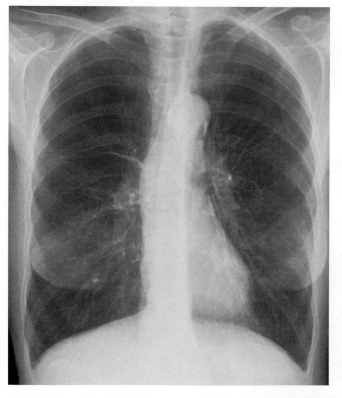

A

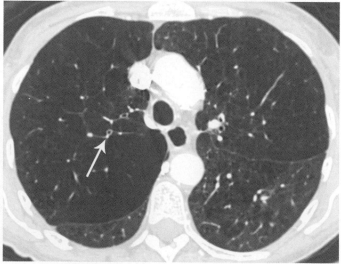

B

Fig. 11.7 (A–C) Emphysema in a 62-year-old woman. **(A)** Chest radiograph demonstrates overinflated lungs, the upper lobes of which appear more lucent than the remainder. **(B)** High-resolution CT of the upper lobes demonstrates severe lung emphysema. A right upper lobe artery is smaller in diameter (*arrow*) than its accompanying bronchus.

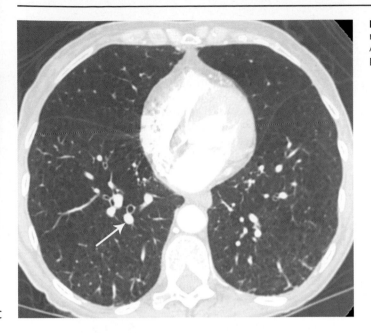

C

◆ Pulmonary Langerhans Cell Histiocytosis

- ◆ Of the patients with this disease, 90 to 100% are current or former smokers.
- ◆ Histologic features include cellular peribronchiolar nodules containing Langerhans cells and inflammatory cells in the early stages. Later, there is a progression from cellular nodules to entirely fibrotic nodules. Adjacent lung changes of respiratory bronchiolitis or desquamative interstitial pneumonitis are common.

- ◆ Pulmonary hypertension in advanced disease is more prevalent and severe than in other chronic lung diseases and appears to be in part due to pulmonary vascular disease.
- ◆ Vasculopathy includes a prominent proliferative inflammation with occasional Langerhans cells involving both arteries and veins.
- ◆ Imaging is characterized by a combination of nodules and cysts, predominantly in the upper and middle regions of the lungs, with sparing of the bases (**Fig. 11.8**).

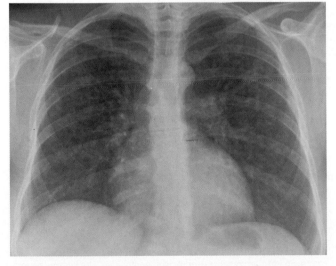

A

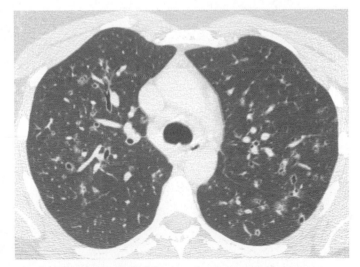

B

Fig. 11.8 (A,B) Pulmonary Langerhans cell histiocytosis in a 35-year-old female smoker. **(A)** Chest radiograph demonstrates numerous bilateral ill-defined nodules, some of which appear cavitary. **(B)** High-resolution CT demonstrates thin-walled lung cysts in the upper lobes as well as small ground-glass nodules. The lung bases were relatively clear.

◆ Usual Interstitial Pneumonitis

- ◆ Usual interstitial pneumonitis is known as idiopathic pulmonary fibrosis when there is no apparent cause.
- ◆ It can be secondary to toxic drugs, environmental exposure (asbestos), or collagen-vascular diseases.
- ◆ The histology includes dense fibrosis causing remodeling of the lung architecture with frequent "honeycomb" change, fibroblastic foci typically scattered at the edges of dense scars and fibrotic zones with temporal hetero-

geneity, and smooth-muscle hyperplasia in areas of fibrosis.
- ◆ In addition to the hypoxia resulting from disease of the lung parenchyma, vascular intimal thickening occurs, which can progress to acellular fibrosis with luminal obliteration.
- ◆ Imaging demonstrates ground-glass attenuation with interlobular septal thickening, architectural distortion with associated traction bronchiectasis and bronchiolectasis, and a honeycomb pattern (**Figs. 11.9** and **11.10**). The

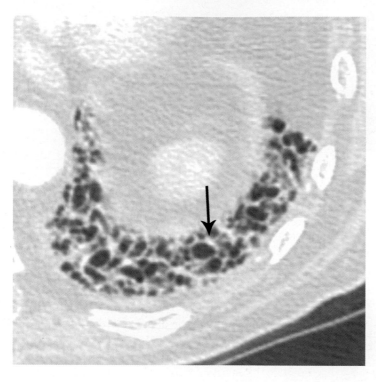

Fig. 11.9 Usual interstitial pneumonitis in a 79-year-old man. High-resolution contrast material–enhanced CT viewed on lung windows demonstrates a pulmonary artery branch within the wall of the honeycomb lung (*arrow*).

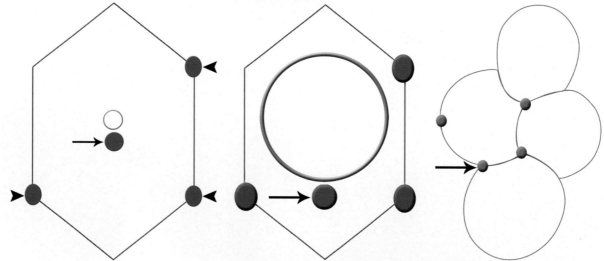

A–C

Fig. 11.10 (A) Illustration of a normal secondary pulmonary lobule. The secondary pulmonary lobule is represented by the *hexagon*; in the center are the bronchiole (*green ring*) and arteriole (*arrow*). In the periphery are pulmonary venules (*arrowheads*). **(B)** Illustration of brochiolectasis. The bronchiole is dilated (*green ring*), and the arteriole is displaced peripherally toward the edge of the secondary pulmonary

lobule (*arrow*). **(C)** Illustration of honeycomb lung. The septa of the honeycomb lung are represented by the *green lines*. The vessels appear smaller and may become occluded and fibrosed (*green circles*). The arteriole has moved from the center of the normal lobule to within the wall of organizing fibrosis of the honeycomb lung (*arrow*).

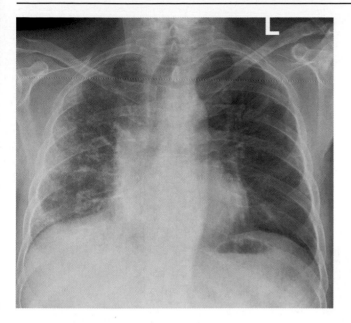

A

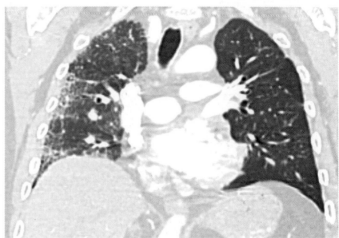

B

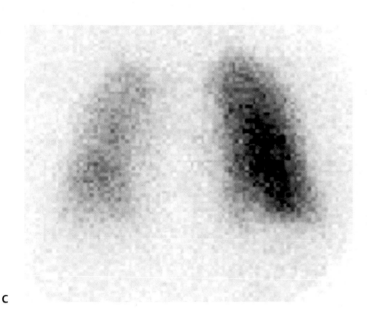

C

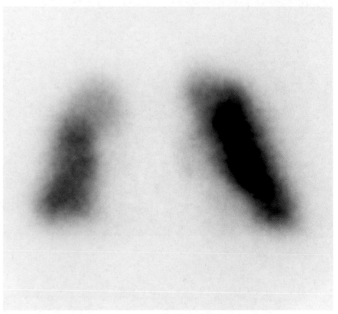

D

Fig. 11.11 (A–D) Left lung transplant in a 64-year-old man with usual interstitial pneumonitis. **(A)** Chest radiograph demonstrates shift of the trachea to the right, indicating right-sided lung volume loss, and the right lung appears to have small reticular-nodular opacities. The left lung appears normal. **(B)** Coronal reconstruction CT demonstrates a small right lung with central and peripheral ground-glass opacification as well as subpleural interlobular septal thickening. The left lung appears normal. **(C)** Xenon 133 ventilation scan demonstrates 39% ventilation in the right lung and 61% ventilation in the left. **(D)** ^{99m}Tc-macroaggregate albumin perfusion scan demonstrates 37% perfusion in the right lung and 63% perfusion in the left.

abnormalities are predominantly basal and peripheral in distribution.

◆ Autoregulation of the pulmonary vasculature causes vasoconstriction in regions of hypoxia, resulting in the preferential perfusion of normal lung (**Fig. 11.11**).

◆ Lymphangiomatosis

◆ Lymphangiomatosis is a congenital abnormality that usually presents in adolescence or early adulthood. It causes dyspnea and wheezing and is easily misdiagnosed as asthma.

- Pathologically, it is characterized by the proliferation of multiple complex lymphatic channels along anatomic lymphatic routes.
- Lymphangiomatosis may involve the lungs and mediastinum, cause lytic bone lesions, and affect other organs.
- It is associated with recurrent chylothorax and pericardial effusions.
- The diffuse compression by abnormal soft tissue on the pulmonary vasculature in the lungs and mediastinum is thought to be a large contributing factor to pulmonary artery hypertension.

- The clinical course varies. In adults, it can be favorable, with a low mortality rate; when the disease presents in children, it is often progressive and relentless.
- Imaging demonstrates pleural and pericardial effusions, smooth interlobular septal thickening, and peribronchovascular interstitial thickening (**Fig. 11.12**). The mediastinum can be affected by a discrete soft-tissue mass or an infiltrative continuum of abnormal soft tissue enveloping the mediastinal structures.

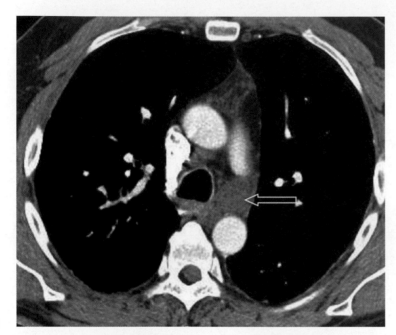

A

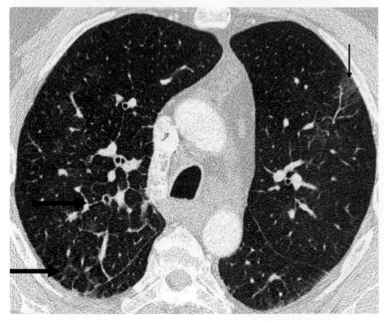

B

Fig. 11.12 (A,B) Lymphangiomatosis in a 48-year-old man. **(A)** CT demonstrates soft-tissue mass in aortopulmonary window (*arrow*). **(B)** CT on lung window settings demonstrates smooth interlobular septal thickening (*thick arrows*) and peribronchovascular interstitial thickening, particularly on the right. There is also bilateral patchy ground-glass opacifications (*thin arrow*). (From El Hajj L, Mazières J, Rouquette I, et al. Diagnostic value of bronchoscopy, CT and transbronchial biopsies in diffuse pulmonary lymphangiomatosis: case report and review of the literature. Clin Radiol 2005;60(8):921–925. Reprinted with permission.)

◆ Capillary Hemangiomatosis

- ◆ Capillary hemangiomatosis is a rare idiopathic cause of pulmonary hypertension that affects the alveolar capillary bed. There is an elevated pulmonary arterial pressure and a normal or low pulmonary capillary wedge pressure.
- ◆ The classic histologic feature is the proliferation of capillary channels within the alveolar walls.
- ◆ Imaging demonstrates widespread ill-defined centrilobular nodules of ground-glass opacity, often mixed with lobular opacities (**Figs. 11.13** and **11.14**).

- ◆ Potent vasodilators (including prostacyclin and calcium channel blockers) can induce florid and even fatal pulmonary edema in patients with capillary hemangiomatosis; if the pulmonary muscular arteries and arterioles are dilated and the pulmonary vein resistance remains fixed, the increased transcapillary hydrostatic pressure leads to the massive transudation of fluid into the lung parenchyma.

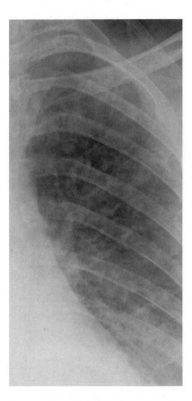

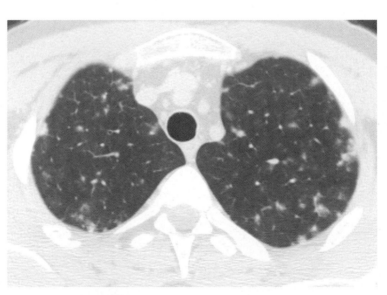

A

B

Fig. 11.13 (A,B) Capillary hemangiomatosis in a 20-year-old man. **(A)** Coned chest radiograph view of left upper lobe demonstrates ill-defined small patches of ground-glass opacification. **(B)** High-resolution CT demonstrates centrilobular and peripheral ground-glass and denser opacities. There is no interlobular septal thickening.

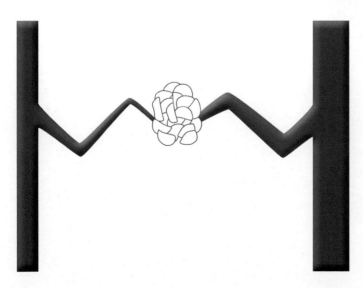

Fig. 11.14 Illustration of capillary hemangiomatosis, represented by the *meshwork of lines* in the center of the picture. The effect is dilation of the afferent pulmonary artery on the right side of the illustration.

◆ Pulmonary Veno-Occlusive Disease

◆ Pulmonary veno-occlusive disease is a rare idiopathic cause of pulmonary hypertension that affects the postcapillary (venous) pulmonary vasculature. There is an elevated pulmonary arterial pressure and a normal or low pulmonary capillary wedge pressure.

◆ Histologically, intimal fibrosis narrows and occludes the pulmonary veins, reducing them from large interlobular vessels to venules of immediate-postcapillary size. Large numbers of veins may be involved, or the process may be patchy.

◆ CT demonstrates ground-glass opacities, which can be centrilobular or panlobular, often with a geographic distribution; additional features are smoothly thickened interlobular septa, pleural effusions, and adenopathy (**Figs. 11.15** and **11.16**).

◆ Prostacyclin and calcium channel blockers are effective treatments for primary pulmonary hypertension; however, these vasodilator therapies can also be very harmful and occasionally fatal in patients with pulmonary veno-occlusive disease.

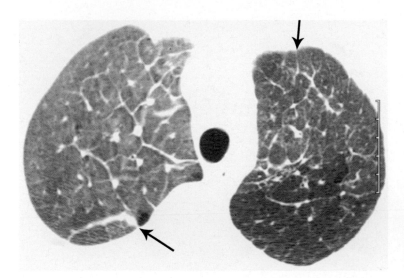

Fig. 11.15 Pulmonary capillary veno-occlusive disease in a 32-year-old woman. High-resolution CT demonstrates prominent smooth interlobular septal thickening (*arrows*), as well as centrilobular or panlobular ground-glass opacities with a geographic distribution.

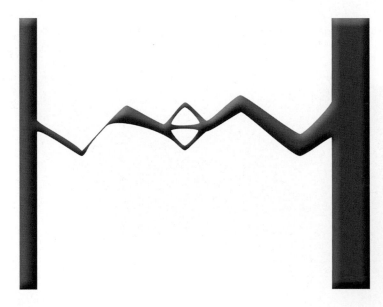

Fig. 11.16 Pulmonary capillary veno-occlusive disease is represented by the obliterated thin vein on the left side of the picture. There is dilatation of the inflowing veins and arteries proximal to (to the right of) the obstruction.

Suggested Reading

Attili AK, Kazerooni EA, Gross BH, Flaherty KR, Myers JL, Martinez FJ. Smoking-related interstitial lung disease: radiologic-clinical-pathologic correlation. Radiographics 2008;28(5):1383–1396, discussion 1396–1398

Barberá JA, Peinado VI, Santos S. Pulmonary hypertension in chronic obstructive pulmonary disease. Eur Respir J 2003;21(5):892–905

Bhalla M, Abboud MR, McLoud TC, et al. Acute chest syndrome in sickle cell disease: CT evidence of microvascular occlusion. Radiology 1993;187(1):45–49

Faul JL, Berry GJ, Colby TV, et al. Thoracic lymphangiomas, lymphangiectasis, lymphangiomatosis, and lymphatic dysplasia syndrome. Am J Respir Crit Care Med 2000;161(3 Pt 1):1037–1046

Frazier AA, Franks TJ, Mohammed TL, Ozbudak IH, Galvin JR. From the Archives of the AFIP: pulmonary veno-occlusive disease and pulmonary capillary hemangiomatosis. Radiographics 2007;27(3):867–882

Girgis RE, Mathai SC. Pulmonary hypertension associated with chronic respiratory disease. Clin Chest Med 2007;28(1):219–232, x

Hennebicque AS, Nunes H, Brillet PY, Moulahi H, Valeyre D, Brauner MW. CT findings in severe thoracic sarcoidosis. Eur Radiol 2005; 15(1):23–30

Howling SJ, Northway WH Jr, Hansell DM, Moss RB, Ward S, Müller NL. Pulmonary sequelae of bronchopulmonary dysplasia survivors: high-resolution CT findings. AJR Am J Roentgenol 2000;174(5):1323–1326

Ioachimescu OC, Sieber S, Kotch A. Idiopathic pulmonary haemosiderosis revisited. Eur Respir J 2004;24(1):162–170

Kinane TB, Westra SJ. Case records of the Massachusetts General Hospital. Weekly clinicopathological exercises. Case 31-2004. A four-year-old boy with hypoxemia. N Engl J Med 2004;351(16):1667–1675

Lee KN, Lee HJ, Shin WW, Webb WR. Hypoxemia and liver cirrhosis (hepatopulmonary syndrome) in eight patients: comparison of the central and peripheral pulmonary vasculature. Radiology 1999;211(2):549–553

Leong CS, Stark P. Thoracic manifestations of sickle cell disease. J Thorac Imaging 1998;13(2):128–134

Resten A, Maitre S, Humbert M, et al. Pulmonary hypertension: CT of the chest in pulmonary venoocclusive disease. AJR Am J Roentgenol 2004;183(1):65–70

Voelkel NF, Cool CD. Pulmonary vascular involvement in chronic obstructive pulmonary disease. Eur Respir J Suppl 2003;46:28s–32s

Wittram C, Mark EJ, McLoud TC. CT-histologic correlation of the ATS/ERS 2002 classification of idiopathic interstitial pneumonias. Radiographics 2003;23(5):1057–1071

Yang DH, Goo HW. Generalized lymphangiomatosis: radiologic findings in three pediatric patients. Korean J Radiol 2006;7(4):287–291

12

Pulmonary Arterial Hypertension

In 2003 in Venice, the World Health Organization adopted a revised classification for pulmonary arterial hypertension (**Table 12.1**).

The majority of the causes of pulmonary arterial hypertension included in the World Health Organization classification have been covered in previous chapters. In this chapter, idiopathic or primary pulmonary hypertension is illustrated as a chronic cause of pulmonary arterial hypertension. In addition, some of the acute causes of pulmonary arterial hypertension and their consequences are illustrated with exercise-induced pulmonary hemorrhage and high-altitude pulmonary edema.

◆ Primary Pulmonary Hypertension

- ◆ By definition, primary pulmonary hypertension is pulmonary arterial hypertension without a known cause.
- ◆ Pulmonary arterial hypertension is defined as a mean pulmonary artery pressure exceeding 25 mm Hg (3300 pascals [Pa]) at rest or 30 mm Hg (4000 Pa) with exercise.
- ◆ The pathologic changes are largely confined to the muscular pulmonary arteries that measure less than 1 mm in diameter. The changes seen in large pulmonary arteries are a response to the pulmonary hypertension.
- ◆ The histologic features range from minor changes of hypertrophy of the muscular media of the small pulmonary arteries to subendothelial fibrous proliferation and "plexiform lesions." These pathologic changes are seen in both primary pulmonary hypertension and pulmonary hypertension with known causes.
- ◆ Radiologic abnormalities include dilatation of the pulmonary arteries (**Fig. 12.1**).
- ◆ As a result of chronically raised pulmonary artery pressure, atheromatous changes may develop in the pulmonary arteries, which can calcify (**Fig. 12.2**).
- ◆ On high-resolution computed tomography (CT), subtle centrilobular ground-glass opacities are often noted (**Fig. 12.1**), which correspond to cholesterol granulomas. These possibly form as a consequence of macrophage ingestion of red blood cells after repeated pulmonary hemorrhage.

Table 12.1 World Health Organization Classification of Pulmonary Arterial Hypertension

Group I. Pulmonary arterial hypertension
Idiopathic (primary)
Familial
Pulmonary arterial hypertension associated with the following:
  Collagen-vascular disease
  Congenital systemic-to-pulmonary shunts (large, small, repaired, or nonrepaired)
  Portal hypertension
  Human immunodeficiency virus infection
  Drugs and toxins
  Other (glycogen storage disease, Gaucher disease, hereditary hemorrhagic telangiectasia, hemoglobinopathies, myeloproliferative disorders, splenectomy)
Pulmonary arterial hypertension associated with significant venous or capillary involvement:
  Pulmonary veno-occlusive disease
  Pulmonary capillary hemangiomatosis
  Persistent pulmonary hypertension of the newborn
Group II. Pulmonary venous hypertension
Left-sided atrial or ventricular heart disease
Left-sided valvular heart disease
Group III. Pulmonary hypertension associated with intrinsic lung disease or hypoxemia
Chronic obstructive pulmonary disease
Interstitial lung disease
Sleep-disordered breathing
Alveolar hypoventilation disorders
Chronic exposure to high altitude
Developmental abnormalities
Group IV. Pulmonary hypertension caused by chronic thrombotic or embolic disease
Thromboembolic obstruction of proximal pulmonary arteries
Thromboembolic obstruction of distal pulmonary arteries
Pulmonary embolism (tumor, parasites, foreign material)
Group V. Miscellaneous causes
Sarcoidosis
Pulmonary Langerhans cell histiocytosis
Lymphangiomatosis
Compression of pulmonary vessels (adenopathy, tumor, fibrosing mediastinitis)

Source: Adapted with permission from Simonneau G, Galie N, Rubin J, et al. Clinical classification of pulmonary hypertension. J Am Coll Cardiol 2004;43(12 Suppl S):5S–12S.

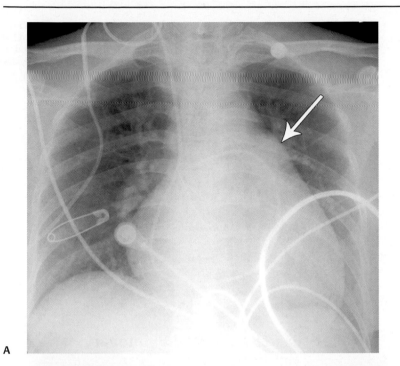

A

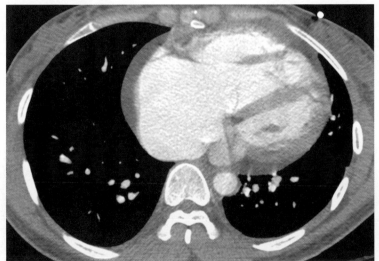

B

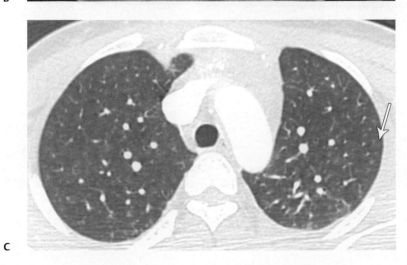

C

Fig. 12.1 (A–D) Primary pulmonary hypertension in a 26-year-old woman. **(A)** Portable chest radiograph demonstrates a heart with a globular shape, a prominent main pulmonary artery (*arrow*), and prominent other pulmonary arteries. **(B)** CT demonstrates dilatation of the right atrium and ventricle as well as a moderately sized pericardial effusion. **(C,D)** High-resolution CT shows that the central pulmonary arteries are much larger than their accompanying bronchi (artery-to-bronchus ratio, >1.2). There are diffuse, ill-defined centrilobular opacities (*arrows*). (*Continued on page 154*)

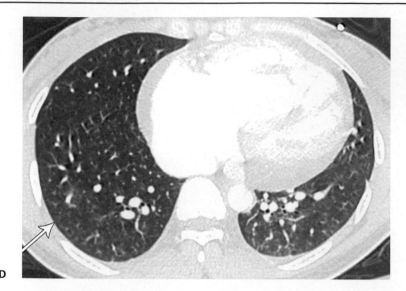

D

Fig. 12.1 (*Continued*) Primary pulmonary hypertension in a 26-year-old woman. **(C,D)** High-resolution CT shows that the central pulmonary arteries are much larger than their accompanying bronchi (artery-to-bronchus ratio, >1.2). There are diffuse, ill-defined centrilobular opacities (*arrows*).

◆ Idiopathic Pulmonary Artery Dilatation

- ◆ This uncommon condition is diagnosed when the main pulmonary artery is much larger than 29 mm in diameter, no cardiac or pulmonary disease is present, and the pulmonary artery pressure is normal (**Fig. 12.3**).
- ◆ A few case reports suggest that the condition is benign and nonprogressive.

◆ Exercise-Induced Pulmonary Hemorrhage

- ◆ It is hypothesized that exercise-induced pulmonary hemorrhage is the result of an acute rise in pulmonary arterial pressure in susceptible individuals engaging in sustained strenuous exercise.
- ◆ This entity is common in racehorses, and cases have been reported in humans (**Fig. 12.4**).

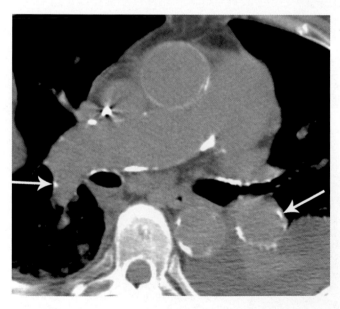

Fig. 12.2 Primary pulmonary arterial hypertension in a 73-year-old woman. Unenhanced CT demonstrates calcifications of the wall of the right and left pulmonary arteries (*arrows*).

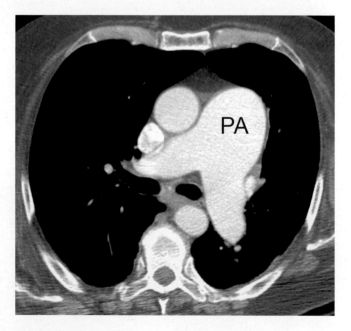

Fig. 12.3 Idiopathic pulmonary artery dilatation in a 66-year-old woman. The main pulmonary artery (*PA*) measured 52 mm in diameter on CT.

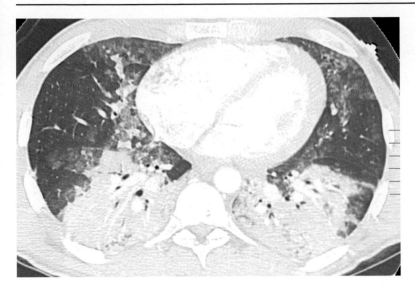

Fig. 12.4 Diffuse pulmonary hemorrhage in a 25-year-old male marathon runner in whom hemoptysis developed during a marathon race in Boston, MA. CT demonstrates bilateral lower lobe consolidation and ground-glass opacities in the middle lobe and lingula, which quickly resolved.

◆ High-Altitude Pulmonary Edema

- ◆ High-altitude pulmonary edema is a life-threatening noncardiogenic pulmonary edema that occurs in otherwise healthy individuals at altitudes above 2500 m.
- ◆ Individual susceptibility is difficult to predict. The most reliable risk factor is previous susceptibility.
- ◆ The pathogenesis includes an increase in sympathetic tone and exaggerated hypoxic pulmonary vasoconstriction, which can be uneven, with increased pulmonary capillary pressure and alveolar fluid leak across capillary endothelium.
- ◆ The radiologic features manifest as central interstitial edema associated with peribronchial cuffing, ill-defined vessels, and a patchy, frequently asymmetric pattern of air space consolidation (**Fig. 12.5**).

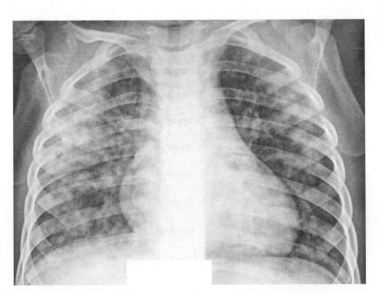

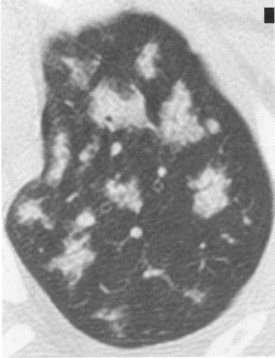

A   **B**

Fig. 12.5 (A,B) High-altitude pulmonary edema in a 10-year-old boy. **(A)** Chest radiograph demonstrates peribronchial cuffing and ill-defined vessels with bilateral ill-defined nodular opacities. **(B)** High-resolution CT of left upper lobe demonstrates ill-defined patches of consolidation. (Courtesy of Dr. S. Martinez-Jimenez.)

Suggested Reading

Ghio AJ, Ghio C, Bassett M. Exrcise-induced pulmonary hemorrhage after running a marathon. Lung 2006;184(6):331–333

Maggiorini M, Mélot C, Pierre S, et al. High-altitude pulmonary edema is initially caused by an increase in capillary pressure. Circulation 2001; 103(16):2078–2083

Nolan RL, McAdams HP, Sporn TA, Roggli VL, Tapson VF, Goodman PC. Pulmonary cholesterol granulomas in patients with pulmonary artery hypertension: chest radiographic and CT findings. AJR Am J Roentgenol 1999;172(5):1317–1319

Ring NJ, Marshall AJ. Idiopathic dilatation of the pulmonary artery. Br J Radiol 2002;75(894):532–535

Simonneau G, Galiè N, Rubin LJ, et al. Clinical classification of pulmonary hypertension. J Am Coll Cardiol 2004;43(12 Suppl S):5S–12S

Tolle JJ, Waxman AB, Van Horn TL, Pappagianopoulos PP, Systrom DM. Exercise-induced pulmonary arterial hypertension. Circulation 2008; 118(21):2183–2189

Ugolini P, Mousseaux E, Sadou Y, et al. Idiopathic dilatation of the pulmonary artery: report of four cases. Magn Reson Imaging 1999; 17(6): 933–937

Index